Ways of Knowing and Caring for Older Adults

Mary Burke and Susan Sherman, Editors

National League for Nursing Press • New York
Pub. No. 14-2541

The views expressed in this publication represent the views of
the authors and do not necessarily reflect the official views of the
National League for Nursing Press.

Library of Congress Cataloging-in-Publication Data

Ways of knowing and caring for older adults / Mary Burke and Susan
    Sherman, editors.
        p.   cm.
    Proceedings of the Second Annual Gerontological Nursing Symposium,
held in San Diego in February 1993: p. 7.
    "Pub. no. 14-2541."
    ISBN 0-88737-593-6 : $29.95
    1. Geriatric nursing—Congresses. 2. Aged—Care—Congresses.
I. Burke, Mary M.   II. Sherman, Susan, RN.
RC954.W29   1993
610.73'65—dc20   93-38938
                                                                CIP

This book was set in Goudy by Publications Development Company
of Texas. The editor was Maryan Malone. The cover was designed by
Lauren Stevens. Clarkwood Corp. was the printer and binder.

Printed in the United States of America

Contents

Contributors

Sister Rosemary Donley, PhD, RN, FAAN
Executive Vice President
The Catholic University of America

Lois K. Evans, DNSc, RN, FAAN
Associate Professor
University of Pennsylvania, School of Nursing
and
Associate Professor and Director
Geropsychiatric Nursing Sub-Specialty

Janet Ikenn Fine, MS, RN, CNAA
Administrator of Health Services
Alexian Village of Milwaukee

Jeanie Kayser-Jones, PhD, RN, FAAN
Professor
Department of Physiological Nursing
University of California

Barbara K. Haight, DrPH, RNC, FAAN
Professor
Medical University of South Carolina

Andrea Mengel, PhD, RN
Professor
Department of Nursing
Community College of Philadelphia

Linda R. Phillips, PhD, RN, FAAN
Professor
University of Arizona

Joanne Radar, RN, MN
Clinical Research Fellow
Benedictine Institute for Long Term Care
Mt. Angel, Oregon

Susan Sherman, MA, RN
National Project Administrator
Community College-Nursing Home Partnership
Professor and Head, Department of Nursing
Community College of Philadelphia

Elaine Tagliareni, MS, RNC
Associate Professor and Project Director
Community College-Nursing Home Partnership
Department of Nursing
Community College of Philadelphia

Holly Skodol Wilson, PhD, RN, FAAN
Professor
Department of Mental Health, Community, and Administrative Nursing
School of Nursing
University of California, San Francisco
and
Affiliated Professor
Aging Health Policy Institute

Preface

The Second Annual Gerontological Nursing Symposium, *Ways of Knowing and Caring for Older Adults*, was held in San Diego in February 1993. The conference was a continuation of the successful, collaborative effort of faculty from the Community College-Nursing Home Partnership Dissemination Project funded by the W.K. Kellogg foundation, Georgetown University Gerontologic Nursing Graduate Program and the National League for Nursing. The success and stimulation of the first conference and its subsequent publication, *Gerontological Nursing: Issues and Opportunities for the Twenty-first Century*, prompted the conference planners of the second symposium to address the fundamental questions of how we as nurses come to know and to care for older adults.

These are exciting and challenging times for gerontological nursing. The issues facing caregivers and educators are complex and continue to grow more pressing. The need to comprehend the basis of gerontological knowledge and the ethic of caring is fundamental to the ability to nurse the elderly client. Nurses, as dedicated providers of care for the frail elderly, are and will continue to be center stage in the debate to define and improve health care for the nation's older adults. Nurses lead the nation in their ability to advocate for the quality of life issues dear to all elderly people.

The papers presented at this conference are outstanding scholarly and experiential papers that address the provocative and challenging issues that face nurses seeking excellence in gerontological nursing. As editors we are indeed grateful to all the authors for their generous spirit, their commitment to gerontological nursing, their uncompromising intellect, and their valued colleagueship.

The papers deal with the tensions of our time: the tensions created by the methodological differences between qualitative and quantitative investigations; the tensions between ways of knowing based on intuitive stories and the ways of knowing from statistical analyses of data; the tensions between innovation and tradition; the tensions between caregivers and regulators; the tensions among health care settings for allocation of health care dollars; and the multitude of tensions that are embedded in human caring relationships. There are no magic solutions but the papers bring new dimensions to the dialogue.

Most significant is the message that addresses the current window of opportunity for gerontological nurses to speak out for adequate and appropriate health care for our nation's elderly population. As we have stated before, this challenge is the moral imperative that must join together all nurses in a common struggle.

The editors wish to thank: Dr. Patricia Moccia, Chief Operating Officer and Executive Vice President, National League for Nursing, for her continued support for gerontological nursing, Dr. Elaine Larson for her commitment to Gerontological Nursing at Georgetown University School of Nursing, Dr. Helen Grace from the Kellogg Foundation for her vision and dedication to the Community College-Nursing Home Projects, Verle Waters for her gracious leadership, and last but not least Allan Graubard, Editor Director, National League for Nursing Press, for his expertise and good humor which brought this book to completion.

Mary (Mickie) Burke DNSc, RN, CANP
Susan Sherman MA, RN

1

Ways of Knowing: Shaping the Chaos

Holly Skodol Wilson

INTRODUCTION

I count as a special honor the privilege of delivering the keynote address for the National League for Nursing's Second Annual Symposium on Gerontological Nursing. I am especially pleased to share the program with so many distinguished colleagues and friends as we discuss, debate, and expand our thinking on "Ways of Knowing and Caring for Older Adults." The eminence of this symposium faculty reminds me of an occasion many years ago when I was watching Saturday morning TV with my youngest daughter, Molly, who was then about 4 years old. "Popeye," a notoriously sexist cartoon, was on, and, much to my pleasure, Molly asked, "Why doesn't Olive Oil try to save herself?" Later she asked, "Why doesn't *she* eat the spinach?" It's such a pleasure for me to participate in a conference that demonstrates what happens when women eat the spinach!

In this presentation, I will explore gerontological nursing's dominant epistemologies, examine contemporary and futuristic conditions that demand a revolution in ways of seeing issues related to improving the

UCSF doctoral student Suellen Miller is gratefully acknowledged for her original contributions to the content of this paper, as is Professor Margarete Sandelowski at UNC.

quality of life and quality of care for the elderly, and advocate a cutting-edge synthesis of humanistic and "new science" modes for investigating and interpreting subjectivity and experience among older adults.

COMPARATIVE EPISTEMOLOGIES IN GERONTOLOGICAL NURSING

Epistemology is the science of the grounds of knowledge. It is the study of assumptions about how to know and apprehend meaning—about that which constitutes valid understanding—and the ways in which we can be sure that we know what we know. It is the study of truth claims. Methodology, on the other hand, is defined as the frameworks on which research is based. Methodological questions have to do with how we can go about finding things out (Fonow & Cook, 1991; Guba & Lincoln, 1989). Questions of methodology are linked to questions of epistemology (Miller, 1992a).

An analysis of nursing research in regard to aging reveals an ongoing tension between two influential paradigms or ways of knowing: the positivist/empiricist and the Naturalistic/Interpretive (Carper, 1978; Miller, 1992a).

The Positivist/Empiricist Paradigm

The positivist/empiricist, "traditional science" paradigm has long dominated nursing's journals and funding agencies. This paradigm, often termed "hard science," holds that:

> Knowledge, composed of facts and principles, exists ahistorically and acontextually as an entity apart from the researcher and the subject. Research conducted under this paradigm adheres to conventions of theory verification and customarily employs quantitative statistical methods derived from the physical sciences. (Miller, 1992a, p. 4)

Here, research follows experimental and quasi-experimental designs, with subject sampling based on probability theory and data collection methods frequently employing standardized instruments, psychometric tests, and questionnaires. The researcher assumes it is possible to find an independently ordered set of facts through rigorously controlled

laboratory experiments. Once discovered, this knowledge, based on random sampling and reliable and valid instrumentation, can be general-
ized to all individuals, regardless of personal meanings and historical
contexts. The goal of positivist research is to control and manipulate
situational variables under experimental conditions. Positivist/empiricist
epistemology allows us to know "that"—allows us to confirm facts scientifically. However, as Patricia Benner (1983) has noted, knowing "that"
is different from knowing "how." Knowing "that" is accomplished
through a unit analysis. Knowing "how" requires a process analysis.
Critics have jokingly dubbed the positivist/empiricist epistemology the
quantoid approach and have viewed our reliance on the so-called hard
sciences as "physics envy." In the grip of this malady, also called method-
idolatry, we come to worship research methods themselves; in such worship, nursing science becomes idolatrous. Dickoff and James, philoso-
phers at Yale University School of Nursing, and their colleagues began
referring to this phenomenon not as physics envy but rather as
"nursing's addiction to pseudo-technical mentality"—a rigid adherence
to what might be inappropriate paradigms for study of nursing's practice
problems under the natural conditions of the real world of clinical care
(Dickoff, James, & Wiedenbach, 1968).

The Naturalistic/Interpretive Paradigm

The naturalistic/interpretive paradigm, by contrast, encompasses such
qualitative designs as discovering, grounded theory, ethnography, and phenomenology. Derived from a belief that research is both historically and
culturally influenced, this research tradition holds that important knowledge can be discovered by studying the interaction between individuals—
including the intersubjectivity between investigator and respondent. This
methodology is comprised of purposive rather than random or probability
samples, and observation and interviews rather than standardized instruments and tests. The naturalistic paradigm uses these processes and methods of data collection and analysis to learn how human experience unfolds
under particular contextual conditions. Naturalistic research allows us to
grasp the hows—the processes of the dailiness of nursing practice—and
is driven by a need to understand rather than a need to control (Allen,
Benner, & Diekelmann, 1986; Wilson & Hutchinson, 1991).

   The dailiness of nursing practice is often fragmented and dispersed,
caught up short among telephone calls, doctors' rounds, patient care orders, and the laundry shortage. It is often episodic and determined by

people and events outside nursing's control. Nurses are continually interrupted. In Bettina Aptheker's (1989) imagery, we carry the threads of many tasks in our hands at the same time. We need to be able to study clinical nursing problems in such a way as to weave a tapestry—a meaningful story—from the threads of feeding, bathing, toileting, feeling, and thinking that make up the dailiness of our everyday practice. Katherine Barnard (1980) has long emphasized the value of case studies. She has pointed out that if we can map out what we learn from one patient—connecting, linking up, weaving together one meaning with another—we can begin to lay out a unique way of seeing reality, a nursing perspective, a middle-range nursing theory that can subsequently inform nursing practice. Dr. Jeanie Kayser-Jones's well-known case study of how a mentally impaired nursing home resident without an advocate was denied appropriate treatment for an acute illness, and ultimately died, is a compelling illustration of the value of case study analysis.

In everyday clinical practice, qualitative analysis is the norm. Each time nonnumerical information is collected about a patient, it must be conceptualized, compared, combined, and categorized to arrive at a clinical interpretation. An elderly patient's self-care capacity, experience of grief, reasons for wandering, and attitude toward mental health care all usually involve more than scores of measurements that can be plotted on a scale and subjected to statistical procedures. Nurse clinicians are experts at grasping the significance of data acquired through observing and talking to patients and families about their subjective experiences. Some call it insight, intuition, or perceptiveness; in fact, it involves some form of qualitative analysis. Without analysis, reading a report of clinical research would be like watching an Andy Warhol movie where an actor did nothing but sleep for eight hours; or, in the case of quantitative research, reading a trunk of computer printouts that typed out the entire data set (something our colleague Dr. Katherine May, now at Vanderbilt School of Nursing, calls "Comprinter Puke-Out").

The lexicon of diverse terminology associated with Naturalistic/Qualitative ways of knowing varies from writer to writer and includes: content analysis, descriptive statistics, quasi-statistics, unstructured methods, induction, grounded theory, discovery methods, theme analysis, coding, categories, field methods, hypothesis generating, ethnomethodology, intersubjectivity, phenomenology, and interpretive research. Regardless of what they are named, Naturalistic/Qualitative approaches are gaining credibility among nurse researchers because of their compatibility with holistic views of patients and nursing.

Positivist/Empiricist knowledge is only one of several ways of knowing. Although the positivist approach denies the significance of subjective experience, nursing's holistic, humanistic practice demands understanding it (Miller, 1992). Naturalistic approaches are based on a conviction that to know *about* people is not enough. Instead, face-to-face interaction is required if we seek the fullest possible comprehension of another's world. Naturalistic/Qualitative research aspires to capture what other people and their lives are about, without preconceiving the categories into which information will fit.

Gerontological nursing needs modes of inquiry and analysis that offer the freedom to explore the richness of human experience with all its variation. Gerontological nursing needs ways of knowing that can verify the order in the experience of aging and can confirm the effectiveness of nursing interventions in patient outcome terms. But gerontological nursing also needs ways of knowing the irregular, the discontinuous, and the erratic sides of the aging experience. No one entrenched epistemology— or methodology, for that matter—in and of itself will lead to advances in gerontological nursing knowledge. True scientific discoveries will probably come only from scientific pluralism. But where chaos begins, classical science stops. Gerontological nursing needs ways to shape the chaos. Our goal is to seek within ourselves ways of recognizing a variety of different voices about the nature and experiences of older adults.

VOICES OF THE ELDERLY

In 1980, 25.9 million people over the age of 65 made up 11.1% of the population. By the year 2000, there will be 36.3 million Americans over 65, or 13.2% of the population. Projections indicate that, by the year 2040, 67.3 million persons, or 20.5%, will be over 65, and, by 2100, 45% of the elderly population will be over 75. An estimated 20% of elders suffer some form of cognitive impairment, and, currently, somewhere between 2.5 million and 4 million Americans are suffering from the ravages of the mind-wasting and personality-robbing affliction called Alzheimer's disease (AD). The incidence of AD is expected to only rise, because people over 85 make up the fastest growing segment of the population. By 2040, the number of cases of dementia in the elderly is likely to reach 7.4 million. In a recent *Journal of the American Medical Association* report, as many as 1 in 10 people over 65—and, astonishingly, nearly half of those over 85—have the disease. We also know that AD is the fifth leading cause of total disability among elders in the United States (Kuhlman, Wilson, Hutchinson, & Wallhagen, 1991).

We know these progressive, orderly trends about the graying of America and the incidence of the Disease of the Century because empirical surveys have enabled us to confirm these objective realities—to study what appears to be predictable and representative of order. These are compelling facts. But, if we listen to the voices that follow, we come face-to-face with the paradox that older adults, while alike in some ways, are different in many others. What ways of knowing can we discover to unmask order in the local, indeterminate, contingent, complex meanings of aging for the expressly divergent group of people we call older adults?

1. Lillian Hellman (1972) offered an image of aging, likening her experience to "pentimento"—a phenomenon that takes place when old paint on canvas becomes transparent, a "way of seeing and then seeing again." She wanted to see what was there for her once and what was there for her in her older years.

2. Meridel Le Sueur (1982) compared the aging human body to an external landscape—each person is marked by the passing seasons, the migrations of people, the "swift turn of a century verging on change never before experienced."

3. Phillip Larkin, in *The Old Fools* (1977), attempted to account for the elderly's "air of baffled absence" by using the metaphor of an internal landscape—the decor of a home. To Larkin, being old is having lighted rooms inside your head and people in them whom you know yet can't quite name; known books from shelves, familiar rooms, and the chairs themselves are trying to be there, yet having to be here.

4. Marion Roach was her mother's voice, when she wrote in *The New York Times* about their experience of early AD:

    In the summer of 1983 my mother killed the cats. We had seven; one morning she grabbed four, took them to the vet and had them put to sleep. She said she didn't want to feed them anymore. It occurred to me that she might be going mad . . . . Day by day she became more disoriented. She would look around at her surroundings as if she had just appeared there. She had difficulty remembering which side of the hall her bedroom was located on. The table with its puzzling array of utensils, plates, and glasses made eating an impossible task. She asked the same questions over and over again, unable to remember she had just said the same thing a few moments before.

My mother, a college graduate who used to say, "Television rots the mind," now spends most of her day watching disco dance shows—literally watching since she rarely turns on the sound—and smoking cigarettes. Until last Fall, she had gone 15 years without a cigarette. Since she can't remember how much she smokes, she smokes about 4½ packs a day. It's one of the few things she remembers how to do.

My mother is 69 years old. She has been a widow for almost 8 years. Soon, within several years, her brain will forget not only what day it is, but how to perform what for most people are automatic functions—how to walk, how to talk—in short, how to live. (Roach, 1983)

5. British poet Jenny Joseph, in "Warning," welcomed the prospect of becoming an old woman, seeing it as an opportunity to wear purple with a red hat that doesn't suit her, to spend her pension on brandy and summer gloves, to sit down on the pavement when she's tired, to gobble up samples in shops, press alarm bells, run her stick along public railings, pick flowers in other people's gardens, go out in slippers in the rain—in short, to "make up for the sobriety of her youth" (Joseph, 1986).

CONDITIONS DEMANDING A "NEW SCIENCE"

In 1987, James Gleick wrote a national bestseller entitled *Chaos: Making a New Science* (Gleick, 1987). Gleick's book on Chaos Theory sketches the history of how newly discovered universal laws about the irregular, discontinuous, and erratic side of nature have been discovered. These laws explain how a falling leaf on some planet in another galaxy might affect the motion of a billiard ball on a pool table on Earth; they tell about the chain of events originally called "The Butterfly Effect," which technically refers to a principle of sensitive dependence on initial conditions.

In natural science, as in nursing, a chain of events can have a point of crisis that can magnify small changes. Chaos Theory added the notion that such points can be everywhere! Research based on the innovative paradigm in the physical sciences has gone on to apply, to the dailiness of life, a revolutionary way of seeing and explaining pendulum clocks, playground swings, horseshoe games, clouds, dripping faucets, fatal arrhythmias, snowflakes, and loaded dice. Chaos has become a shorthand name for a fast-growing movement that is reshaping the fabric of the scientific establishment because chaos:

- Breaks across lines that separate scientific disciplines and is a holistic rather than reductionist approach.
- Looks for patterns in complexity and what appears as randomness.
- Has spawned a new language of "fractals," "bifurcations," "intermittencies," "periodicities," and "smooth noodle maps."
- Has made everyday experience in the real world the legitimate target for inquiry.
- Has recognized the need to account for the fact that order and chaos can occur together because our world is one of nonlinearity. Order masquerades as randomness.

Chaos has become the century's third great revolution in the physical sciences. Relativity eliminated the Newtonian illusion of absolute space and time. Quantum theory eliminated the dream of a controllable measurement process. Chaos eliminates the fantasy of deterministic predictability.

Are there similar paradigm shifts taking place in the social, behavioral, and caring sciences that may offer a way of knowing about the holistic, divergent, complex, nonlinear discontinuities reflected in the voices and stories of America's older adults?

POSTMODERNISMS: TOWARD A "NEW SCIENCE" OF GERONTOLOGICAL NURSING

Philosopher Kenneth Burke once said, "A way of seeing is also a way of not seeing." Critics of the dominant paradigms of Positivist/Empiricist and Naturalistic/Interpretive human science argue the need for paradigms that, like Chaos Theory in physics, go beyond objectivism versus relativism and acknowledge that both paradigms have represented ways of *not* seeing certain complexities. They urge us to move into more contemporary debates about knowledge claims. They challenge us to look in our science for the multiplicities, indeterminancies, fragmentations, and pluralities in small-scale situated knowledge. These pluralities of culture, tradition, values, and ideologies are not arranged according to evolution or hierarchies, nor are they categorized as correct or incorrect. Knowledge of them must occur in the context of the culture and language/symbols that make them possible and endow them with meaning. Postmodern epistemologists hold that neither truth nor wholly objective knowledge is to be gained by any particular standpoint. They believe that truth is a historical product and that knowledge is socially constructed. They posit that, in the world of human experience, there is only interpretation. Attempting to make interpretation available to others is a worthwhile goal because, by so doing, understanding can be created. They believe in the value of questioning or "deconstructing" monolithic concepts like truth, knowledge, power, the self, and language—all of which have been taken for granted as foundational enlightenment beliefs. They feel that, to some extent, such transcendent knowledge claims reify the experience of a few White, Western males. Among the foundational beliefs being challenged, questioned, and deconstructed by poststructural, postmodern thinkers are these (Miller, 1992):

1. That knowledge acquired by reason will be true, universal, and unchanging and will reflect an objective reality—something "out there" independent of the knower and not created in the mind of the knower.

2. That history is progressive and reasonable, that events are not random, and that there is a rational structure, comprehensible by reason alone, to why events occur.

3. That reason is transcendent and universal and that science as the height of reasoning is the preferred paradigm for all knowing.

In short, poststructuralist postmodernisms refer to specific forms of cultural critiques that have emerged in intellectual circles since the mid-1970s. These critiques, according to Miller (1992) refuse the appeals of epistemological absolutes. They view long-proclaimed notions of the enlightenment's Western social order as partial, foundationalistic, contingent, and historically situated. The concepts of postmodernisms are often worded in neologisms and jargon. In running down the list of jargon in postmodern discourse, sociologist Elvi Whittaker commented that that list alone allows her to look back on the writings of Talcott Parsons with some degree of nostalgia (we in nursing might have the same reaction to the language of someone like Martha Rogers). She also went on to ask the 1991 Stone Symposium audience, "What is a postmodern mafia?" The answer: "One that makes you an offer you can't understand." Despite the opinion of some who say that to be positioned within the domain of "modernity" is merely the latest form of verbal abuse, postmodern thinking has gained recognition in philosophy, anthropology, sociology, political science, history, theology, and psychology, and in the "hard" sciences: Chaos Theory, subatomic physics, and fractal geometry. Little evidence of postmodern thinking and theorizing, however, has appeared in the nursing literature to date. A computer search revealed 5 articles, all of which agree that, from a postmodern position, there is no Archimedean standpoint from which to view "reality" and that any understanding of reality is a representation, not a mirror of nature (Miller, 1992).

Postmodern epistemologists would probably agree with Lily Tomlin when she says, in her search for intelligent life in the universe, "Reality is no more than a collective hunch." They would ask us to consider the notion that it is impossible to describe the elderly under one theory without doing damage to significant differences among people. They would urge us to listen to these words of a 66-year-old African American, lesbian, feminist, socialist mother of 2, and member of an interracial couple:

> I usually find myself a part of some group defined as other, deviant, inferior, or just plain wrong. It's not our differences that separate us. It's our refusal to recognize these differences and to examine distortions that result from misnaming them and their effect on human behavior and expectation. It's a lifetime pursuit for each one of us to examine these distortions from our living and at the same time recognize, reclaim, and define those differences imposed on us. (Miller, 1992a)

Postmodern perspectives offer gerontological nurse clinicians and researchers the opportunity to look beyond surface similarities of a mythical elder's voice to study the wide-ranging diversity of experience real people have.

Postmodern epistemology allows for a multiplicity of positions, acknowledging the contradiction implicit in them and accommodating ambiguity.

Postmodern epistemology speaks in terms of heterogeneity—a language that privileges no single point of reference.

Postmodern epistemology encourages us to indulge in multiple paradigms and to question their underlying assumptions of what research is, who it is for, and what effects the findings will have on those who have been studied. Postmodern studies are conducted under the rubric of feminism, critical social theory, and interpretive interactionism.

Postmodern epistemology allows us to understand how people make sense of their lives—struggling personally and collectively for meaning in a complex, changing, and often chaotic world. Elders are not understood as "essential core identities" but rather as persons in process, situated in culture and time, constructing themselves and being constructed by others (Miller, 1992).

TOWARD A SYNTHESIS OF HUMANITIES AND "NEW SCIENCE"

There is no doubt that we live in a time of profound epistemological skepticism and methodological soul searching (Miller, 1992). Our faith in the claims of science to truth and objectivity has, over the past 20 years, been shaken by the rediscovery of the subjective nature and "storied" quality of science (Sandeslowski, in press). Physicists draw parallels between modern quantum physics and oriental mysticism, write about intuition's role in both, and conclude that both the dancing God and physical theory are creations of the mind; they are models to describe their authors' intuition of reality.

Nisbet (1976), a sociologist, talked about the oxymoron of participant observation, where we strive for a cool but not cold detachment from a warm but not hot engagement with the subjects/informants/respondents/participants of our studies and assert yet deny our own signature voice—our authorial presence in the findings of our studies. Like Lillian Hellman, we claim to be both there—a part of what we studied, and here—appropriately removed from it. We are confronted with the problem of making science out of biography, theory out of lives. Poststructuralist/Postmodern thought points out, "Our work is located now on the faultline presumed to exist between art and science" (Sandelowski, in press).

Scientific and artistic approaches are believed by some to differ in their aims, sources of data, forms of representation, and criteria for appraisal. Yet the kinship of art and science can be affirmed in their mutual beginnings and in the creative act.

The word *theory* comes from the same Greek roots as the word *theater*. In sociologist Nisbet's view, a tragedy or a comedy is, after all, no less an inquiry into reality, no less a distillation of perceptions and experiences than a hypothesis or theory that accounts for the variable incidence of marriage or murder (Nisbet, 1976).

What we must strive for is not a science devoid of its art, but rather a science with the spirit of discovery and creation left in. Both the scientist and the artist are concerned with illuminating reality, exploring the unknown, and creating and peopling worlds. Often, artistic truths when compared with scientific ones provide us with visions of human nature that are more resonant with our own experience. In the words of my colleague and friend, Margarete Sandelowski:

> The greatest fictional characters from Shakespeare's Hamlet to Ibsen's Nora are those who though not existing in real life, still reveal recurring or dominant human tendencies; the secrets of the human heart that we have shared and with which we can readily identify. . . . Even widely fanciful departures from camera truth in paintings (consider Picasso or Dali's work) may in part be in the service of fidelity to its subject matter. Language, after all, is itself like a work of art—selecting, abstracting, exaggerating, ordering. In neither science nor art does language signify things as they are but rather as they are perceived as being by the observer. (Sandelowski, in press)

Science cannot claim truth, rigor, or explanation solely for itself, and art cannot claim beauty, imagination, and poetic license solely for itself. Again, according to Sandelowski, "Whether we are motivated by impulses to make our work scientific or artistic, we still make it up."

Every good investigator in the world has to take a sudden leap, to be good at what she or he does. Without that leap, we remain mere fact grubbers and rule followers. Celebrating art permits adding nonscientific sources of knowledge (literature, art, music, dance) to frame and enhance our understanding. The elders of the next decades won't be singing "Let Me Call You Sweetheart"; they will have been the Woodstock Generation, who listened to The Doors. We must learn about them in a way that is phenomenologically true to the people and events in their lives, and hermeneutically self-conscious of the methods and interests in our research. Sandelowski once wrote:

> I have always been drawn to research papers that look more like finely crafted romances than lab reports. I am drawn to a research report that tells a good story, but is also aesthetically and intellectually satisfying. I have only lately realized that I never aspired to be a scientist, but rather

a certain kind of writer. When you ask me about my research, don't ask me what I found. I found nothing. Ask me what I invented from my data. But know that in asking you to ask me this, I am not confessing to telling lies. I have told the truth. The proof for you is in the stories I have made; how they look to your mind's eye; whether they satisfy your sense of style and craftsmanship, whether you believe them, whether you come to know something important because of them and whether they appeal to your heart. (in press)

CONCLUSION

Early in this paper, I shared some metaphors writers have used to portray the experience of aging. I'd like to end with a fable adapted from Ingram (1988) to portray something important about the diversity of our ways of knowing.

In the beginning, the All-Knowing planted a garden. In the midst of the garden, She placed the Tree of Knowledge. This tree produced a veritable fruit salad, with many different kinds of fruit growing on each of its branches. There were apples and oranges, kumquats and pears, peaches, bananas and plums, and more. And each contained the seeds of a different type of knowledge. To the visitors who wandered into the garden, the All-Knowing said, "You may eat of the fruit of the Tree of Knowledge." The visitors who ate the fruit became known as researchers, and came and went from the garden as they pleased, or as their federal grants or top budgets allowed.

One day, a visitor strolled to the Tree and inquired about the various fruits growing there. The All-Knowing pointed to a small group of researchers who had just finished eating a shiny, red fruit. "These persons have just sampled the Empirical Apple, a tart and somewhat dry fruit, which is currently quite abundant. It opens the mind to the wonders of the senses—sight, sound, touch, taste, smell—and induces an overpowering urge to measure the known universe." As the visitor watched, the "Empiricists," as they were called, scurried about with watches, rules, thermometers, blood pressure cuffs, and calculators, looking very serious and mumbling a good deal to themselves about p. values and statistical significance.

"What is that fruit?" asked the visitor as she pointed to a star-shaped crystal at the tree's summit.

"That," replied the All-Knowing, "is the fruit of Practice Theory. It used to grow on a peripheral branch, but Dickoff and James moved it to the top of the Tree. It looks pretty good there, don't you think?" The visitor agreed and asked what it tasted like.

"Not many people know," sighed the All-Knowing. "Those who are most interested in Practice Theory are the clinic nurses who come here after working double shifts. They usually manage to climb to the middle branches, then fall asleep." As She spoke, several nurses in crumpled white uniforms began ascending the Tree. "Let's hope that they get farther than they did last time."

The visitor spied a small group of researchers lying beneath the Tree, crunching loudly on long, woody objects. "Who are they?" she asked. "Those are the Grounded Theorists. The fruit that they seek is actually a root, or a series of roots, that grows beneath the Tree. The roots synapse with other roots, creating an underground network that spans the entire garden. The researchers spend a lot of time eating roots, partly because they are so hard to digest and partly because of their addictive effect." As the visitor watched, the Grounded Theorists tasted the roots, looked perplexed, and asked aloud, "But what's the Basic Social Process?"

Another group of researchers wafted by, holding fruits that changed color and shape when passed from one person to another. They spoke in muted voices and empathetic tones, and they sighed frequently. "What kind of fruit is that?" enquired the visitor. The All-Knowing smiled. "That is the fruit of Phenomenology. It never appears entirely the same to anyone at any particular time. To one fellow, it is blue and soft; to another, it is green and spiky. Those who eat it become very tolerant of others' opinions, produce copious notes, talk about novices and experts, and wander in and out of an existential vacuum for weeks at a time."

Finally, the visitor came upon an exotic-looking fruit with a green skin that looked much greener than any other fruit in the vicinity. "I think I'd like to try this." "A fine choice," the All-Knowing commented. "That is called the Ethnographer's Delight. You'll find its taste quite unusual." The visitor gingerly bit into the fruit and was overcome with the urge to finish it elsewhere, preferably in another culture. "Thanks for the tour," she said, munching the fruit and eyeing the horizon.

The All-Knowing watched the visitor scurry away. Dusk was falling on the garden and another day was nearing an end. The Empiricists hurried home to their computers to analyze the data that they had collected. The clinicians in search of Practice Theory descended wearily from the Tree's middle branches, and promised to return on their next day off.

The Ethnographers were off to a sale on Birkenstocks, and the Grounded Theorists were engaged in a tug-of-war with the resident sociologists over the various roots. The Phenomenologists muttered, "But what is the meaning of it all?" And the All-Knowing smiled.

REFERENCES

Allen, D., Benner, P., & Diekelmann, N. (1986). Three paradigms for nursing research: Methodological considerations. In P. L. Chinn (Ed.), *Nursing research methodology: Issues and explanation* (pp. 23–38). Rockville, MD: Aspen.

Aptheker, B. (1989). *Tapestries of Life*. Amherst: The University of Massachusetts Press, 1989.

Barnard, K. E. (1980). Knowledge for practice: Directions for the future. *Nursing Research, 29*, 208–12.

Benner, P. (1983). Uncovering the knowledge embedded in clinical practice. *Image: The Journal of Nursing Scholarship. 15*(2), 36–41.

Carper, B. A. (1978). Fundamental patterns of knowing in nursing. *Advances in Nursing Science, 1*(1), 13–23.

Dickoff, J., James, P., & Wiedenbach, E. (1968). Theory as a practice discipline: Part 1—practice-oriented theory. *Nursing Research, 17*, 215–235.

Fonow, M. M. & Cook, J. A. (1991). Back to the future: A look at the second wave of feminist epistemology and methodology. In M. M. Fonow & J. A. Cook (Eds.), *Beyond methodology: Feminist scholarship as lived research* (pp. 1–15). Bloomington: Indiana University Press.

Gleick, J. (1987). *Chaos: Making a new science*. New York: Viking.

Guba, E. G., & Lincoln, Y. S. (1989). *Fourth generation evaluation*. Newbury Park, CA: Sage.

Hellman, L. (1972). *Pentimento*. Boston: Little, Brown & Co.

Ingram, M. R. (1988). Origins of nursing knowledge. *Image: The Journal of Nursing Scholarship, 20*(4), 233.

Joseph, J. (1986). *Persephone*. Newcastle upon Tyne: Bloodaxe Books.

Kuhlman, G., Wilson, H. S., Hutchinson, S. A., & Wallhagen, M. (1991). Alzheimer's disease and family caregiving: Critical synthesis of the literature and research agenda. *Nursing Research, 40*(6), 331–337.

Larkin, P. (1977). *The less deceived*. London: Marvell Press.

Le Suer, M. (1982). *Ripening: Selected work 1927–1980*. Old Westbury NY: Feminist Press.

Miller, S. (1992a). *Methodological issues in a feminist nursing Research Study of New Mothers' Career Re-entry*. Unpublished paper, University of California at San Francisco.

Miller, S. (1992). *Understanding fractured identities: Postmodern feminist perspectives for nursing research on career women and mothering.* Unpublished paper, University of California at San Francisco.

Nisbet, R. (1976). *Sociology as an art form.* New York: Oxford University Press.

Roach, M. (1983). Another name for madness. *The New York Times,*

Sandelowski, M. (in press). "The proof is in the pottery." In J. Morse, (Ed.), *Issues in qualitative research.* Newbury Park, CA: Sage.

Wilson, H. S., & Hutchinson, S. A. (1991). Triangulation of qualitative methods: Heideggerian hermeneutics and grounded theory.

2

Ways of Knowing: Research in Gerontological Nursing

Jeanie Kayser-Jones

Nursing care of the elderly is provided daily in thousands of acute, chronic, and long-term care settings. Much of that care, however, is not based on scientific research, and therein lies the challenge for gerontological nurses. Only through the collaborative efforts of clinicians and research investigators will nurses be able to improve the quality of care for older adults.

This paper first presents some statistics because, when discussing gerontological nursing research, we must examine the issue within the demographic, political, and economic context of our society. Next are the research priorities in aging that have been identified by a committee of the Institute of Medicine (1991). The recommendations of this committee will certainly influence the direction of future research, and it is important for nurses to lead and to be a part of the research teams that will investigate these significant problems.

A brief history of gerontological nursing research is followed by a discussion of some current research programs, including research that I have

The research reported was supported by a grant from the National Institute on Aging (NIA #AG05073).

been conducting for the past ten to fifteen years. Finally, suggestions for future research are presented, and the role of nurses in shaping the research agenda is discussed.

NUMBER AND PROPORTION OF ELDERLY

The care of the elderly is one of the most important and perhaps one of the most controversial issues in health care today. The increase in the number and proportion of older people throughout the world is a major success story of the latter part of the 20th century. But the success that has been achieved presents health care professionals with formidable challenges (Kayser-Jones, 1992).

In the United States, 12% of the population is 65 years and older. This percentage will change very little—from 12% to only 13%—between now and the year 2005. The absolute number of old people, however, will rise from 29 million to 36 million during the same time period. As the post-World War II baby boom matures, the percentage of elderly in the United States will increase from 13% in 2005 to nearly 20% in 2025. At that time, it is estimated that there will be 59 million elderly people in the United States (U. S. Department of Commerce, Bureau of the Census, 1987).

The Oldest Old

In a relatively recent, but very important demographic trend, more people are living to very old age—that is, 80 years of age and older. This group of people, commonly referred to as the "oldest old" is now and will most likely continue to be the fastest growing age group in the United States as well as in other developed and developing countries.

In 1985, the United Nations estimated that nine countries (China, India, The United States, the former Soviet Union, Japan, Brazil, Indonesia, the Federal Republic of Germany, and Italy) had over 1 million people who were 80 years of age and over. The countries with the most octogenarians were: the United States with 6,198,000, China with 5,697,000, and the former Soviet Union with 4,610,000 (U. S. Department of Commerce, Bureau of the Census, 1987).

Most older persons are vigorous, have a good quality of life, and enjoy increasing life expectancy, but chronic diseases do occur and have become a major cause of death and disability. Many of these chronic diseases, such as arthritis, heart disease, and stroke, lead to disability, decline, and dependency in old age.

Another important social factor is the rapidly increasing cost of health care. In 1965, the United States spent $41.6 billion on health care. By 1975, health care expenditures had risen to $133 billion. In 1990, expenditures were a massive $671 billion (more than 11% of the gross national product), and it is projected that, in the year 2000, health care expenditures will reach $1,615.9 billion (Health Care Financing Administration, unpublished data).

Because of the increase of chronic illness in old age, it is not surprising that the amount of health care costs per person is significantly higher for older people. In 1987, per-capita spending for personal health care for those under the age of 65 was $1,286; for those over the age of 65, it was $5,360. Per-capita spending for those 85 years of age and over was 2½ times that for people who were 65–69 years of age (Waldo, Sonnefeld, McKusick, & Arnett, 1989).

The urgent need to respond to the increased number and proportion of elderly, along with the increasing cost of health care, is underscored even further by the fact that the population of those 85 years of age and over is growing six times faster than the rest of the population—and these people are the most vulnerable to physical and cognitive disability (Institute of Medicine, 1991).

The United States has begun to realize the social and economic consequences of the rapidly increasing number and proportion of elderly. For example, the National Institute on Aging was established in 1974. Numerous academic programs in gerontology and geriatrics have been established in nursing and medical schools, and there has been a great increase in research activity into the problems of old age.

Despite the tremendous increase in research activity, however, our scientific knowledge in the field of aging lags far behind what is needed to address the problems of old age.

FUTURE RESEARCH NEEDS IN THE CARE OF THE ELDERLY

Recognizing the tremendous need for research in aging, in 1988, the Institute of Medicine (IOM) convened a committee of eighteen national authorities on health care to identify research priorities on age-related problems for the next twenty years.

Four teams had expertise in these areas: (1) basic biomedical research; (2) clinical research; (3) social and behavioral research; and (4) health services delivery research. Two national authorities in the field of biomedical ethics assisted the committee. Among the 66 experts in health care who comprised these teams, there was only one nurse, Dr. Patricia Archbold, from the Oregon Health Sciences University.

Basic Biomedical Research

Two research priorities were identified by the Basic Biomedical Research group: (1) research in abnormal cell proliferation, and (2) the aging brain. The first priority, abnormal cell proliferation, would investigate the fundamental process responsible for the appropriate replacement of cells that are lost either because of exposure to toxins or because of endogenous physiological processes. Abnormal cell proliferation plays a major role in several of the most important age-related disorders—cancer, atherosclerosis, osteoarthritis, benign prostatic hyperplasia, and altered immune function (Martin, 1979). The second research priority, the aging brain, would focus on basic research in the neurosciences, including the peripheral and central nervous systems. This would include, for example, basic research on Alzheimer's disease.

Clinical Research

In the area of clinical research, two priorities were identified: (1) functional impairment and disability, and (2) the interaction of age-dependent physiological changes and disease.

The first priority, research into the causes, prevention, management, and rehabilitation of functional disability in the elderly is of tremendous importance, and it is an area in which nurses could play an extremely important role. In 1985, the National Health Interview Survey found that 23% of all elderly people were unable to perform at least one of the activities of daily living (ADLs), such as bathing, dressing, and grooming (National Center for Health Statistics, 1985).

About 50% of those who are 85 and older need assistance in performing one or more ADLs and in carrying out one or more instrumental activities of daily living (IADLs), such as shopping, cooking, managing finances, and using public transportation.

When the elderly are no longer able to perform ADLs or IADLs, they become dependent. It is estimated that 1 million to 1.5 million elderly people who live in the community or in an institution are unable to carry out 5 or more ADLs (Branch, Kneidmann, & Papsidero, 1984). Recent studies, however, indicate that these deficits may respond to rehabilitation, thus changing a person's status from dependency to independence.

In some elderly people, functional dependency is associated with one or more specific geriatric clinical syndromes. Geriatric syndromes represent a cluster of symptoms, conditions, and disabilities that result in a variety of physiologic changes and pathological and comorbid conditions.

Several of these syndromes—failure to thrive, impaired postural stability, strength and mobility, urinary incontinence, and mismanagement of medications—are areas that are particularly ripe for research (Institute of Medicine, 1991).

Behavioral and Social Research

The first research priority identified by the behavioral and social research group was the investigation of the basic social and psychological processes of aging, and the specific mechanisms that underlie the interrelationships among social, psychological, behavioral, and biological aging functions. It is well known that there is tremendous variation in how individuals age. One person who is 85 may be institutionalized with severe physical and cognitive disability; another 85-year-old may be a vigorous person living independently in the community. Research is needed that will investigate the interrelationship among the social, cultural, psychological, and physiological variables that influence health, longevity, functional ability, and well-being.

The second priority in this area is research that addresses the issue of population dynamics. Forecasting the number and proportion of older people in future decades and estimating the proportion of those people who will be able to live independently is an important area for investigation.

The third priority identified by the social and behavioral scientists is research that investigates how changes in the social structure of our society will affect the process of aging. For example, how will family structure, retirement policies, and the changing role of women in our society affect the process of aging?

When doing research, special attention should be given to ethnic and racial minorities and to older women who may be adversely affected by social factors such as employment, financial status, or lack of access to health care.

Health Services Delivery Research

The United States has made enormous advances in the area of biomedical research, but our existing health care system for the elderly can best be described as chaotic, fragmented, inadequate, and poorly distributed.
    In this area, the committee identified the following 5 research priorities:

1. Research on long-term care and continuity of care for the elderly.
2. Research on the cost and financing of health care for the older population. Research is needed, for example, that will investigate how financial barriers to care can be eliminated, especially in the areas of mental health, rehabilitation, and long-term care.
3. Research on drug therapy, that is, how certain drugs affect the social and physical functioning of older people, and how drugs can be prescribed and dispensed efficiently and effectively.
4. Research on mental health services for the elderly.
5. Recommended research on disability/disease prevention and health promotion among the elderly.

Research in Biomedical Ethics

Ethical issues abound in all aspects of health care for older people. The research priorities identified in this area are:

1. Research on decisions regarding life-sustaining treatment. We need to investigate, for example, how to improve the decision-making process for cognitively impaired people who have not given clear advance directives.
2. Research on equity and access to health care. Should age, for example, be a criterion that is used to limit or withhold treatment?
3. Research on the ethical issues investigators face when conducting clinical research on frail or cognitively impaired elderly. For example, people with severe dementia cannot give consent to

participate in clinical studies, yet there is a need to conduct research on patients with dementia (Institute of Medicine, 1991).

A BRIEF REVIEW OF GERONTOLOGICAL NURSING RESEARCH

Having presented research priorities, I would like to turn now to a brief discussion of research that has been conducted in the past by gerontological nurses. In the past twenty-five years, extensive reviews of gerontological nursing research have been published (Adams, 1986; Basson, 1967; Brimmer, 1979; Cora & Lapierre, 1986; Gunter & Miller, 1977; Haight, 1989; Kayser-Jones, 1981; Murphy & Freston, 1991; O'Leary, McGill, Jones, & Paul, 1990; Robinson, 1981; Wolanin, 1983).

The first review, by Basson (1967), examined selected gerontological literature from 1955 to 1965. Basson found that, of 438 articles reviewed, 372 were not directly related to research. Of the remaining 66 articles, only 12% could be classified as research papers.

Gunter and Miller analyzed studies in *Nursing Research* from 1952 to 1976. Interestingly, during this twenty-four year period, only seventeen papers on the elderly were published; 5 were clinical studies, 4 were papers that focused on attitudes of nursing staff and students, and 8 were surveys of the characteristics and problems of the aged. Of all the review authors, only Gunter and Miller reviewed non-nursing literature. In reviewing the psychosocial literature, they found twenty-nine studies, of which 9 were on the psychosocial characteristics, 4 investigated attitudes of nursing personnel, and 16 were on nursing interventions for the elderly.

Future reviews should include studies that are published in non-nursing journals such as *The Gerontologist, Journal of the American Geriatric Society,* and *Social Science and Medicine.* Increasingly, nurses are publishing in such journals. Some attempt should be made to review research that appears in non-nursing journals, although this may be somewhat difficult because authors are not always identified by their professional titles. Perhaps the task could be facilitated by obtaining the names of nurses who belong to the Gerontological Society of America. In 1991, 1,015 nurses (15% of the membership) belonged to this organization. If these nurses were contacted and asked to submit a bibliography, a more comprehensive review could be conducted.

Kayser-Jones (1981b) surveyed the five nursing journals most likely to report research. *Western Journal of Nursing Research, Research in Nursing* and Health, Journal of Gerontological Nursing, and Geriatric Nursing were reviewed from their beginning dates of publication through July 1980. Gunter and Miller had reviewed Nursing Research through 1976, so I reviewed this journal from January 1977 to July 1980. Forty-four research articles were found: twelve had a clinical focus, 7 were on the attitudes of health professionals toward the elderly, 9 dealt with the psychosocial problems of the aged, 7 focused on the problems of the institutionalized aged, 3 on health needs of the elderly in the community, 2 on human sexuality and aging, 2 on minority aging (specifically, on African American elderly), and 2 were review articles.

I concluded that, although there had been a gradual increase in gerontological nursing research, it was limited in scope and depth, and there were no large-scale, well-defined research programs that systematically investigated the promotion, maintenance, and restoration of health for the elderly (Kayser-Jones, 1981b). An important point of this review was the educational context of nursing students. At this time, I proposed that the lack of geriatric and gerontological nursing content in basic nursing educational programs contributed to a lack of preparation of a cadre of nurses at the graduate level who were educated and thus able to conduct gerontological nursing research.

Wolanin (1983) published a review of clinical research in geriatric nursing. She organized the papers according to clinical issues such as research on personal care, sleep problems, medications, the effect of polypharmacy, movement therapy and how it affected the morale and self-esteem of the aged, and incontinence. Interestingly, although incontinence is a major problem that should be of great interest to nurses, Wolanin found that the studies of it, with one exception (Catanzaro, 1981), were at least fourteen years old.

Wolanin (1983) also discussed the conceptual and methodological problems in conducting clinical geriatric nursing research. The first conceptual issue discussed was the lack of a consistent definition of old age. Some investigators define old age as those who are 65 years of age or older; others include people who are only 55.

Adams (1986) noted that investigators did not distinguish between subjects who are 65 and those who are 95. She proposed that sampling and data analyses should be based on the young old (65 to 74 years), the middle old (75 to 84), and the old old (85 years of age and over). With more and more people living to 85 years and older, investigators must take this problem into consideration when designing future research studies.

The second conceptual issue discussed by Wolanin was: "Who represents the aged?" She noted that most research has been conducted on the elderly who are convenient, such as those in congregate housing or in nursing homes. There has been little research on the care of the elderly in the home and in acute care settings.

Other conceptual concerns were (Wolanin, 1983): Are the right questions being asked and investigated, or are only the easy questions being studied? Are nurse researchers investigating the concerns that have high priority for clinicians and that will contribute to a higher quality of care for the elderly? Do the conceptual issues that are being studied, such as incontinence and caregiving, lead to theory development?

Several reviewers noted that most early research studies did not originate from a conceptual or theoretical base. Murphy and Freston (1991) analyzed gerontological nursing studies from 1983 to 1989 to determine the extent to which theory was combined with research. They found that, although there has been considerable growth in theoretically based studies, many studies did not generate or test theory.

Several reviewers have discussed methodological problems: the lack of replication studies, the need for longitudinal rather than cross-sectional studies, the limitations of questionnaires in obtaining data from elderly, the lack of research on minority elderly, sampling problems, and the fact that most research has been focused on disease and disability. There is concern, for example, that we will present an erroneous picture of old age if we study only the elderly who are accessible because they are easily ill; we are then ignoring the healthy elderly, who may be playing golf, climbing mountains, or engaged in numerous creative and intellectual pursuits.

EXAMPLES OF CURRENT PROGRAMS OF RESEARCH

In the later years of the 1980s and the early 1990s, there has been a tremendous growth in the gerontological nursing research literature. As the number of gerontological nursing programs has increased, there has been a correspondingly higher number of nurse investigators, and they have become increasingly successful in obtaining research grants from federal agencies and private foundations.

An important recent trend is the growth of programs of research that study important, clinically relevant problems that have direct application to practice. Among them are: Bergstrom's and Braden's research on the prediction and prevention of pressure sores (Bergstrom & Braden, 1992; Bergstrom, Braden, Laguzza, & Holman, 1987; Bergstrom, Demuth, & Braden, 1987; Braden & Bergstrom, 1987); the research of Wells, Brink, Diokno, Wolfe, and Gillis (1991) on urinary incontinence; and Strumpf and Evans's work on the use of restraints (Evans & Strumpf, 1992; Strumpf & Evans, 1988; Strumpf, Evans, Wagner, & Patterson, 1992).

Bergstrom and Braden, for example, have developed the Braden Scale, which can be used by clinicians to predict the risk for pressure sore development (Bergstrom, Braden, et al., 1987). Pressure sores are a significant problem, and nurses have struggled for years to prevent and treat them. The work of these investigators has important implications for nurses in acute and long-term care facilities as well as for home care nurses.

Dr. Thelma Wells's research on urinary incontinence is well known by nurses in academia and clinical practice (Wells, et al., 1991). Urinary incontinence is a major clinical problem that affects at least 10 million adult Americans (U. S. Department of Health & Human Services, 1988). Yet, when Dr. Wells began her research program in 1982, there was virtually no research being done in this area. Wells and her research group have found that pelvic exercises are beneficial in reducing stress incontinence, the most common cause of urine leakage reported by older women living in the community. Wells's work is an excellent example of how knowledge obtained from research can be utilized in clinical practice.

The use of physical restraints is another extremely important clinical problem, and Drs. Lois Evans and Neville Strumpf have been pioneers in conducting research that addresses this issue. Their early work powerfully and poignantly described, from the patients' perspective, what it is like to be restrained when hospitalized. One patient, for example, said, "I felt like a dog and cried all night. It hurt me to have to be tied up. I felt like I was nobody, that I was dirt. It makes me cry to talk about it. The hospital is worse than a jail" (Strumpf & Evans, 1988).

In a study of two long-term care facilities in Scotland and Sweden that, combined, accommodated 460 residents, these researchers found that no restraining devices were used at either facility, with the exception of one seat belt that a resident had requested (Strumpf, Evans, Williams, & Williams, 1991). These findings are in sharp contrast to those in the United States, where over 40% of residents in skilled nursing facilities are regularly restrained in chairs and beds.

Evans and Strumpf have found that education is a critical element in changing the nursing staff's beliefs about restraint use (Strumpf, Evans, Wagner, & Patterson, 1992). The findings of their research have incredibly important implications for clinical practice.

Of a different nature, but equally important, is the work of Dr. Charlene Harrington, one of the most influential and distinguished investigators in the area of health policy research. Her current project, titled, "Home Health and Nursing Home Market Analysis," examines state policies, socioeconomic condition, and other factors that affect the supply and demand for nursing home and home health care. A recent article by Harrington and her colleagues provided the first trend data on state nursing home occupancy rates in the United States (Harrington, Preston, Grant, & Swan, 1992). The findings of Dr. Harrington's research are in great demand by policymakers, and using the results of her research, on numerous occasions, she has testified before legislative bodies at the state and federal levels. This brief review only touches on the sophisticated and important research that is being done today by gerontological nurses.

I will now describe how my research has evolved from a small-scale, single-investigator research project to a much larger interdisciplinary research program.

KAYSER-JONES'S RESEARCH PROGRAM: A DEVELOPMENTAL PERSPECTIVE

In describing my research career trajectory, I hope to illustrate several important points. First, research careers, for many of us, are developmental. Many nurses begin their research careers by conducting small-scale, single-investigator studies. Very few nurses who currently have successful research programs started out as principal investigators on large, multidisciplinary research projects.

Second, investigators do not always begin with clear, well-defined research goals. Many factors influence one's choice of research topics; serendipity often plays a role. Third, the more one learns when conducting research, the more one begins to realize the magnitude and the complexity of the research problem. One question leads to another, or one answer leads to another question. Then comes the realization that no one person has the knowledge, skill, and ability to find the answers to complex research questions. And this, in turn, leads to building a research team.

Fourth, with the development of an interdisciplinary research team, one soon learns that productivity increases and the quality of work improves. It just proves the old adage: Two heads *are* better than one.

In looking back, I realize that my research career actually began in the mid-1970s, when I was teaching undergraduate nursing students in a baccalaureate program. Several of my students were working in nursing homes, because, as they told me, they could always find employment there. They insisted that, when they graduated, they would never work in a nursing home.

I was puzzled by their comments and discussed this situation with a colleague in the Department of Psychology. We decided to conduct a research study in which we would investigate nursing students' interest in working with elderly patients. We found that students at all levels (freshman, sophomore, junior, and senior) showed minimal interest in working with the elderly (Kayser & Minnigerode, 1975).

When I conducted that first research project, I did not have a doctoral degree, and I had no plans for entering a doctoral program. In teaching clinical nursing, however, I often came upon clinical practice questions that cried out for answers, and, in 1976, I entered a doctoral program in medical anthropology at the University of California, Berkeley. At that time, I became very interested in the care of the institutionalized elderly. This was somewhat surprising to me because, like many nurses, I had always worked and taught in acute-care hospitals.

Two factors were responsible for this new interest. First, Dr. Margaret Clark, a professor at the University of California, San Francisco (one of the founders of the medical anthropology program), was a distinguished gerontologist, a pioneer in the field of anthropology and aging, had published a book, Culture and Aging, that was highly regarded, and was an inspirational mentor.

Second, my grandfather, whom I admired and loved very much, died in a nursing home. At the time of his death, I was a young head nurse working in a major teaching hospital. Then, as is common today, I was one of the many health care professionals who believed that everything important in health care revolved around major acute-care facilities. Although I had been a nurse for several years, I had never been inside the doors of a nursing home.

One evening, my mother called to tell me that my 94-year-old grandfather, because of failing health, had been placed in a nursing home. I went home that weekend to visit him. I was aware of a depressing environment and unpleasant odors as I entered the building and walked down the hallway to the room where my grandfather lay. The drapes were drawn; the room was quiet and darkened as if waiting for death's approach.

I stood by my grandfather's bed and spoke to him; he did not reply. His eyes were closed, and his demeanor was that of a person who had lost hope. This was so unlike my grandfather, who had been an extremely strong and independent man all of his life, that I could hardly believe he was the same person. Leaning over the bedside rail, I took his hand in mine, kissed him goodbye, and left the room, knowing that I would not see him again. He died that night.

In the intervening years, when I read or heard about the poor conditions in nursing homes in the United States, my thoughts often went back to my beloved grandfather. Thus, it is not surprising that ten years later, when I considered various topics for research, I chose to focus on the care of the institutionalized elderly.

When reviewing the literature on the care of the elderly, prior to beginning my doctoral dissertation research, I learned that in the United Kingdom there was an organized system of health care for the elderly. The National Health Service Act of 1946 had made it possible to promote geriatrics as a new specialty in medicine (Brocklehurst, 1975). The National Health Service provided a structure for the organization and financing of the British Geriatric Service, an innovative approach to long-term care.

As a young anthropologist, I believed it would be valuable to do a cross-cultural comparative study of one long-term care institution in Scotland and one in the United States. As a doctoral student, I was the sole investigator. The study focused on comparing the quality of care in the two institutions, attempting to identify the factors that contributed to a high quality of care (1981a). This study, published as a book titled *Old, Alone, and Neglected: Care of the Aged in Scotland and the United States* (Kayser-Jones, 1981c), was important in launching my career in gerontology and gerontological nursing.

In subsequent years, building on my doctoral research, I conducted several small studies aimed at understanding further the dynamics of institutional life and how to improve the quality of care in nursing homes.

As I continued to work in nursing homes in the early 1980s, I became aware that nursing home patients often became acutely ill. Some were sent to a hospital for treatment; others remained in the nursing home. Some of these patients recovered, and some died.

I was beginning to see many articles in the medical, nursing, and social science literature that focused on the increasing number and proportion of elderly people and the profound effect they would have on the utilization and cost of health care services.

There was controversy in the literature as to whether the elderly should be treated aggressively when they became acutely ill. Most of the articles focused on the clinical, ethical, legal, and economic problems faced by physicians, patients, and their families in deciding whether to treat or withhold treatment.

One article by a physician, in *The New England Journal of Medicine* (Hilficker, 1983), had a profound effect on me. The doctor poignantly described how difficult it was for him to decide whether he should treat or withhold treatment for a nursing home resident, a woman he had known for many years when she had lived independently in her home. Now, after several strokes, she was in a nursing home with contractures, physical disability, and cognitive impairment. She had developed pneumonia, and he recounted the thoughts that went through his mind as he drove to the nursing home to see her and to make a decision regarding treatment.

Although there was an extensive body of literature on the social, ethical, and legal issues of treatment or nontreatment, I found that there had been no prospective studies that had systematically investigated the treatment of acute illness in nursing homes.

I applied for a research grant to investigate the social, cultural, and clinical factors that influence decision making in the treatment of acute illness in nursing homes. In 1985, I received a 3-year grant from the National Institute on Aging to investigate this problem. When I was writing the grant application, I realized that my days of being a lone investigator were over, and I put together an outstanding research team to assist me: a full-time project director, a physician/geriatrician, a quantitative analyst, and 6 research assistants.

We followed 215 nursing home residents who became acutely ill, and described in detail the treatment and management of their acute illness. We also interviewed doctors, nursing staff, residents, and their families (100 persons in each category), to record their attitudes and beliefs regarding the treatment of acute illness.

While collecting data for this study, several independent observations collectively led to the development of our next research project. First, we found that nursing home residents sometimes became severely dehydrated and were sent to an acute care hospital for rehydration therapy. One woman was so dehydrated that, when she arrived at the acute care hospital, the doctor found that her tongue was literally stuck to the roof of her mouth.

Second, we observed that many residents did not eat well. In two of the nursing homes in which we were collecting data, the nursing staff reported that 50–60% of the residents had some problem with eating. In some cases, when residents lost a significant amount of weight because they were not eating well, nasogastric feeding tubes were inserted (Kayser-Jones, 1990b).

Third, when interviewing the residents, we did not ask their opinion about the food. At the end of the interview, however, we did ask: "How do you feel about your life here in the nursing home?" Interestingly, in response to this question, food was often the first concern mentioned. Most of the residents were very dissatisfied with their meals; only two made favorable comments. Complaints about the food centered around three issues: (1) the unpleasant features of the dining room; (2) the manner in which meals were served, and (3) the poor quality of the food.

Fourth, when interviewing families, we found that they, too, were unhappy with the food that was served, and some were concerned about the manner in which residents were being fed by the staff. An interview of the mother of a young man who had received a severe head injury in an automobile accident led to another interesting piece of information. When this young man was admitted from the acute care hospital to the nursing home, he was being fed with a nasogastric tube. The mother observed that her son was able to swallow his saliva. "I thought," she said, "that if he could swallow his saliva, he could also swallow food." She therefore, asked the nurses if they would try feeding him, but they refused her request, saying that he would choke. She then asked if she could feed him. Her son was being cared for on a large multibed ward. The nurses said that if she wanted to feed him, she could do so, but she would have to take him off the ward because they did not want to be held responsible if he should choke while being fed.

It was a long, tedious process, but eventually the mother was able to feed her son adequately and the feeding tube was removed. Interestingly, only family members and one of the nursing assistants were successful in feeding this young man.

This observation was of great interest to me and raised some important questions: Why was the mother able to feed her son successfully? Why were the nurses unwilling to try to feed him? As I reflected on these observations, I began to realize that, during the years of conducting research in nursing homes, food, the mealtime environment, and eating/feeding problems had repeatedly emerged as important issues in institutional life.

In the Scottish–American study, for example, food was identified as an important aspect of care. The Scottish residents were pleased with their food and commented on the pleasure they derived from choosing items from a selective menu. By comparison, the American residents complained about the poor quality of the food, the lack of a selective menu, the absence of fresh fruits and vegetables, and the unpleasant environment at mealtime (Kayser-Jones, 1990a).

It appeared that food and the mealtime environment were significant problems; yet, in reviewing the literature, we found that there had been very little research on eating/feeding problems among the elderly in the United States. I designed my next planned study: "The Behavioral Context of Eating and Nutritional Support." Its purpose will be to investigate eating problems and the use of feeding tubes in nursing homes. The major focus will be to examine the problem contextually, aiming to unravel the multiple social, cultural, clinical, and environmental factors that influence eating and contribute to the placement of feeding tubes.

In this study, we will interview nursing home residents, their families, doctors, and nursing home staff (75 persons in each category), and we will prospectively follow 100 residents who have an eating problem. This project will require a larger research team than the previous study. I will be the principal investigator and there will be a full-time project director. A physician/geriatrician will do a medical evaluation of residents with eating problems; a doctor of pharmacy will provide pharmacological expertise as to the effects of medications on eating behavior; a dentist will assist us in doing an oral health assessment; a doctorally prepared dietitian will help us do a nutritional analysis of a subsample of the 100 residents with eating problems; two statisticians will oversee and direct the quantitative data analysis; a speech pathologist will do a bedside dysphagia evaluation when the physician deems it necessary; and we will have a total of 4 research assistants to assist in data collection.

As you can see, my research program has not been as focused as that of Dr. Wells, who has conducted research on urinary incontinence, or that of Dr. Bergstrom, who has focused on pressure sore prevention.

During the past fifteen years, quality of care, the nursing home environment, and the culture of the nursing home have been the conceptual frameworks within which my research has been grounded. Theoretically, my research has been based in several theoretical frameworks, including, for example, social exchange theory, distributive justice, decision-making theory, and, currently, labeling theory.

Within these broad conceptual areas, I have focused on numerous problems and issues such as bathing, grooming, and elimination (Kayser-Jones, 1981b); room accommodations (Kayser-Jones, 1986); factors that contribute to the hospitalization of nursing home residents (Kayser-Jones, Wiener, & Barbaccia, 1989); advocacy for the mentally impaired elderly (Kayser-Jones & Kapp, 1989); the use of nasogastric feeding tubes in nursing homes (Kayser-Jones, 1990b); ethical decision making (Kayser-Jones, Davis, Wiener, & Higgins, 1989; Kayser-Jones, 1993b); the use of restraints (Kayser-Jones, 1992b), and environmental factors that contribute to falls (Kayser-Jones, 1993a).

A Conceptual Model

Over the years, my research has led to the development of a conceptual model that I believe is useful for both researchers and clinicians. This conceptual model has been used to analyze data in a study that I conducted on falls in nursing homes (Kayser-Jones, 1993a) and in another on the use of restraints (Kayser-Jones, 1992b).

While conducting my research in nursing homes, I have become very interested in the nursing home environment. Broadly speaking, the environment is defined as everything that surrounds us—the neighborhood we live in, the people with whom we interact, the air we breathe, and the design of the buildings in which we live and work. Most research has focused on four features of the environment: (1) the physical characteristics, (2) the organizational climate, (3) the personal and suprapersonal environment, and (4) the social–psychological milieu (see Figure 2.1).

The physical characteristics of a nursing home include, for example, the architectural design, color, lighting, type of floor surface, and space (the size of residents' rooms). The organizational aspects are items such as policy, patient/staff ratio, financing, and nursing and medical leadership. The personal environment concerns those who constitute the major one-to-one relationships of an individual—typically, family, friends, and

Figure 2.1
The Environment: A Conceptual Model for Research and Practice

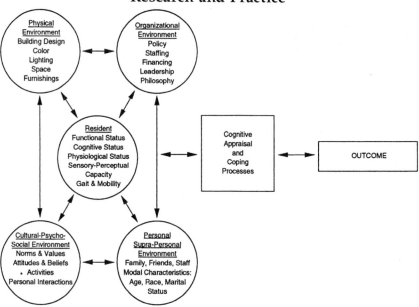

colleagues. In the nursing home setting, a resident's personal world may also be made up of family and friends, but the nursing home staff often constitute a major part of his or her personal world.

The suprapersonal environment is defined as the modal characteristics of all the people who are in physical proximity to an individual. In the nursing home, the modal characteristics of residents in physical proximity to one another include people who are typically very old (85 or older), have multiple physical, functional, and cognitive impairments, and suffer from 3 to 5 pathological conditions such as heart disease, cancer, Parkinson's disease, and stroke. The cultural–social–psychological milieu refers to the norms, values, and philosophy of the administration, and the attitudes and beliefs of the caregivers and residents.

In Figure 2.1, the two-way arrows between circles illustrate that factors in one component of the environment may interact with elements in another and, individually or cumulatively, they may have an effect on the nursing home resident. For example, if the dining room is crowded, noisy, and poorly lighted, the physical environment may affect how residents eat. Similarly, if staffing requires one nursing assistant to feed 8 to 10 residents within a limited time period, the amount of food eaten may be small.

Factors in the personal/suprapersonal area may also affect how residents eat. In our pilot study, for example, we observed that residents often ate better when they were fed by family members, and that some residents would eat for one nursing aide but not for another. The attitudes and beliefs of the caregiver may also affect eating behavior. A caregiver who values older people and believes they deserve to be treated kindly may be more patient and thus successful in feeding a resident. On the other hand, if a caregiver believes that people who need to be fed are uncooperative and undeserving, he or she may be unsuccessful in feeding a resident.

In the center of this environmental system, elderly people—many with cognitive, functional, and sensory-perceptual impairment, and with multiple pathologies (for which they may be taking several medications)—are placed. It is a new and strange environment, frequently devoid of friends, family, personal belongings, and favorite foods. An important component of this model is how each person appraises and then copes with or responds to the various environmental factors.

One could hypothesize, for example, that if the dining room is comfortable and nicely decorated, the staffing ratio is such that each staff member has only one or two residents to feed, and the caregivers treat residents with dignity and respect while feeding them, the elderly person appraises the situation and eats well. If the converse of all of this occurs, however, one could hypothesize that the resident will eat poorly.

This model, I believe, is useful for research and practice because, if we can identify environmental factors that affect eating behavior, an intervention study could be designed to test hypotheses.

Similarly, nurse clinicians could use this conceptual model to assess the environment of a health care setting, attempting to identify factors that may contribute to eating problems, to the use of restraints, or to a high incidence of falls.

FUTURE RESEARCH ISSUES

A great deal of progress has been made; however, there is still an enormous need for gerontological nursing research in the future. The areas for research will be presented under three broad categories: (1) research that will keep the elderly healthy, active, and as independent as possible; (2) research that will focus on equal access to health care when illness does occur; and (3) research that will focus on acute, rehabilitative, and chronic continuing-term care needs of the elderly.

I am sure we would all agree that keeping the elderly healthy, active, and independent is an important goal. To achieve this aim, educational programs that enhance the knowledge, motivation, and skills of the elderly are needed. The importance, for example, of exercise, proper nutrition, and elimination of habits (such as smoking) that are harmful to one's health could be the focus of educational programs that are initiated and later evaluated by nurse investigators. Research demonstration projects that focus on primary health care could be implemented and evaluated by nurse investigators.

Despite the best efforts, unfortunately, illness will occur. One of the greatest problems in the United States is lack of access to health care, especially for certain groups such as the minority elderly and the poor. Descriptive studies of neglected populations, their health care needs, and the problems that arise when health care services are not available are critically needed. Cross-cultural studies that describe and analyze how health care is provided in other countries may be the first step toward finding a solution to our problems. Although the United States has made enormous contributions to health care nationally and internationally, we have a great deal to learn from other countries about the delivery of health care services.

With the Clinton Administration in Washington, I am optimistic about the future. The social and economic problems in the United States, however, are enormous, and these problems may have a negative effect on the elderly. For example, in a recent issue of *Newsweek* it was noted that two-thirds of the major American corporations either have curtailed or will curtail health care plans for retirees in 1993. This action could affect about 10 million elderly people.

Companies, in an attempt to cut costs, are reneging on past promises to their workers. One man, for example, who retired in 1987 after 34 years with a company was told that he would have to pay only $5 a month for a retiree health plan. In 1992, he was told that he would have to pay $144 per month, and that his wife would have to pay $326 a month (Beck & Cohen, 1993). For many of the elderly, this increase would be a serious financial burden, making it impossible for them to continue to pay for their health plan, and thus limiting their access to health care.

There is a tremendous need for research on the acute, rehabilitative, and continuing-care needs of the elderly. We know very little about what happens to elderly people who enter acute-care facilities. Why do many become cognitively impaired and functionally disabled during hospitalization, and could these problems be avoided?

Fulmer and Walker in their book, *Critical Care Nursing of the Elderly*, noted that there has been no substantial nursing research to guide practice in critical-care geriatrics, despite the fact that 50% of all inpatient acute-care admissions in the United States are for people over the age of 75 (Fulmer & Walker, 1992, p. 3).

There is a great need for research on prescribed drugs and the critically ill older patient, and on acute confusional states. Studies that evaluate the advantages and disadvantages of medical and surgical intensive care of the elderly are essential to providing care that is ethical and of a high standard. These studies will be increasingly important as health care costs continue to rise and there is increasing competition for resources. Today, there is great concern about overtreating the elderly. I, however, am concerned that treatment will be withheld solely on the basis of age, or mental status, especially in the home, where decisions are often made by one person (typically, a physician) without consultation with others.

Nurses could make a tremendous contribution by conducting research on rehabilitation. Rehabilitation research is, for the most part, still in its infancy; observational studies that identify problems and describe current rehabilitation practices would be invaluable (Carr, 1991).

Another area that offers nurses a rich opportunity for research is home care of the elderly, the fastest growing segment of health care today. More and more people are being cared for at home, for a number of reasons:

1. As mentioned earlier, more people are living to a very old age, and this group often has multiple chronic illnesses and disabilities that require services.

2. Hospitals are discharging people earlier, or, as the saying goes, "quicker and sicker." Consequently, many people need home care following discharge.

3. Increasingly, patients are being sent home with technological devices that previously were used only in the hospital. We have entered an era where patients are sent home with treatments such as total parenteral nutrition, dialysis, and intravenous antibiotics. Yet, we have very little data as to how patients and their families cope with these complex therapies.

In the fall of 1992, I participated in a study titled "The Technological Tether," funded by the Commonwealth Foundation. It was my first experience in conducting research on home care. I was shocked when I saw the condition in which patients were being discharged, often with little preparation and sometimes with inadequate follow-up.

One of the problems in identifying research priorities is that social conditions and health care needs can change so rapidly that it requires constant vigilance and tremendous energy from all of us, to keep abreast of the most urgent needs. It is imperative that nurse scientists and nurse clinicians work together to identify these needs and design studies that will address the problems and subsequently provide a scientific basis for practice.

Gerontological nursing research—the systematic inquiry into the health, illness, and care of the aged—is of tremendous importance of all of us who are concerned with the alleviation of the problems of old age. The goal of gerontological nursing research is to provide a scientific basis for the practice of gerontological nursing and ultimately to provide optimal care for the elderly in the home, in the community, and in all types of institutional settings (Kayser-Jones, 1981b).

Nurses practice in all of these settings, and they are responsible for providing care and coordinating health care services twenty-four hours a day. Nurses, therefore, are in a position to provide a unique perspective on the health care needs of the elderly and future research priorities.

In 1991, Dr. Thelma Wells received the Sigma Theta Tau International Baxter Foundation Episteme Award. When receiving this award,

Dr. Wells said that an interactive, circular relationship encompasses the domains of practice, research, and education. Research questions come to us from clinical practice, which leads to the development of research projects and new knowledge. The new knowledge is conveyed via education and utilized in clinical practice. Higher-level questions emerge from practice, and the cycle begins again, spiraling ever upward toward excellence in nursing care. This description of the interrelationship between practice and research beautifully illustrates the theme of this conference, "Ways of Knowing and Caring for Older Adults." Knowing is the process of discovering the unknown; through research, we will find the answers to the problems that abound in gerontological nursing. Only when those answers are found will we be able to care for the elderly in a scientific, humane, and ethical way.

As I continue to work with the elderly, my thoughts often go back to a beautiful woman whom I met in a nursing home several years ago. She asked if I were married. She then told me that she and her husband had been married for over 50 years. "I hope that you and your husband will be as happy as we have been," she said. "But we have lived too long. I am too old to take care of him, and he is too old to take care of me."

The challenge for all of us is to find ways of knowing and caring for the elderly so that there will be someone there to care for them when they can no longer care for themselves or each other.

REFERENCES

Adams, M. (1986). Aging: Gerontological Nursing Research. In H. Werley, J. J. Fitzpatrick, & R. L. Taunton (Ed.) *Annual review of nursing research* (pp. 77–103). New York: Springer.

Basson, P. H. (1967). The gerontological nursing literature search: Study and results. *Nursing Research 16*, 267–272.

Beck, M., & Cohen, A. (1993, January 11). Big costs, broken promises. *Newsweek*, p. 59.

Bergstrom, N., & Braden, B. (1992). A prospective study of pressure sore risk among institutionalized elderly. *Journal of the American Geriatric Society, 40*, 747–758.

Bergstrom, N., Braden, B., Laguzza, A., & Holman, V. (1987). The Braden Scale for predicting pressure sore risk. *Nursing Research, 36*(4), 205–210.

Bergstrom, N., Demuth, P. J., & Braden, B. J. (1987). A clinical trial of the Braden Scale for predicting pressure sore risk. *Nursing Clinics of North America, 22*(2), 417–428.

Braden, B., & Bergstrom, N. (1987). A conceptual schema for the study of the etiology of pressure sores. *Journal of Rehabilitation Nursing, 12*(1), 8–12, 16.

Branch, I. G., Kniedmann, K. K., & Papsidero, J. A. (1984). A prospective study of functional status among community elders. *American Journal of Public Health, 74,* 266–268.

Brimmer, P. (1979). The past, present and future in gerontological nursing research. *Journal of Gerontological Nursing, 5*(1), 27–34.

Brocklehurst, J. C. (1975). Great Britain. In J. C. Brocklehurst (Ed.), *Geriatric care in advanced societies.* Lancaster, England: MTP.

Carr, E. K. (1991). Observational methods in rehabilitation research. *Clinical Rehabilitation, 5,* 89–94.

Cora, V. L., & Lapierre, D. (1986). ANA speaks out . . . research in gerontological nursing. *Journal of Gerontological Nursing, 12*(6), 21–26.

Catanzaro, M. (1981). "Shamefully different": A personal meaning of urinary bladder dysfunction. In M. Batey (Ed.), *Communicating nursing research* (Vol. 14). Boulder, CO: Western Interstate Commission for Higher Education.

Fulmer, T. T., & Walker, M. K. (1992). *Critical care nursing of the elderly.* New York: Springer.

Gunter, L., & Miller, J. (1977). Toward a nursing gerontology. *Nursing Research, 26,* 208–221.

Haight, B. K. (1989). Update on research in long-term care: 1984–1988 IN: *Indices of quality in long-term care: Research and practice.* New York: National League for Nursing.

Harrington, C., Preston, L., Grant, H., & Swan, J. (1992, Summer). Trends in nursing home bed capacity in the United States. *Health Affairs.*

Health Care Financing Administration. (Office of the actuary; data from the Office of National Health Statistics.) Unpublished data.

Hilficker, D. (1983). Sounding board: Allowing the debilitated to die—facing our ethical choices. *The New England Journal of Medicine, 308,* 716–719.

Institute of Medicine. (1991). *Extending life, enhancing life.* Washington, DC: National Academy Press.

Kayser, J. S., & Minnigerode, F. A. (1975). Increasing nursing students' interest in working with aged patients. *Nursing Research, 24*(1), 23–26.

Kayser-Jones, J. S. (1981a). A comparison of care in a Scottish and a United States facility. *Geriatric Nursing: American Journal of Care for the Aged, 2*(1), 44–50.

Kayser-Jones, J. S. (1981b). Gerontological nursing research revisited. *Journal of Gerontological Nursing, 7,* 217–223.

Kayser-Jones, J. S. (1981c). *Old, alone and neglected: Care of the aged in Scotland and the United States.* Berkeley: University of California Press.

Kayser-Jones, J. S. (1986). Open ward accommodations in a long-term care facility: The elderly's point of view. *The Gerontologist, 26,* 63–69.

Kayser-Jones, J. S. (1990a). *Old, alone and neglected: Care of the aged in the United States and Scotland.* With a new epilogue. Berkeley: University of California Press.

Kayser-Jones, J. S. (1990b). The use of nasogastric feeding tubes in nursing homes: Patient, family and health care provider perspectives. *The Gerontologist, 30*(4), 469–479.

Kayser-Jones, J. S. (1992a). The acute care of the elderly in the United States: A nursing perspective. *Hong Kong Journal of Gerontology, 6*(1), 4–12.

Kayser-Jones, J. S. (1992b). Culture, environment, and restraints: A conceptual model for research and practice. *Journal of Gerontological Nursing, 18*(11), 13–20.

Kayser-Jones, J. S. (1993a). Influence of the environment on falls in nursing homes: A conceptual model. In R. Kane, M. Mezey, & P. Katz (Eds.), *Advances in long term care* (Vol. II). New York: Springer.

Kayser-Jones, J. S. (1993b). Surrogate decisions for nursing home residents. In G. Winslow & J. Walker (Eds.), *Facing limits: Ethics and health care for the elderly.* Boulder, CO: Westview Press.

Kayser-Jones, J. S., Davis, A., Wiener, C. L., & Higgins, S. (1989). An ethical analysis of an elder's treatment. *Nursing Outlook, 37*(6), 267–270.

Kayser-Jones, J. S., & Kapp, M. (1989). Advocacy for the mentally impaired elderly: A case study analysis. *American Journal of Law and Medicine, 14*(4), 353–376.

Kayser-Jones, J. S., Wiener, C. L., & Barbaccia, J. C. (1989). Factors contributing to the hospitalization of nursing home residents. *The Gerontologist, 29*(4), 502–510.

Martin, G. M. (1979). Proliferative homeostasis and its age-related aberrations. *Mechanisms of Aging and Development, 9*, 385–391.

Murphy, E., & Freston, M. S. (1991). An analysis of theory-research linkages in published gerontologic nursing studies. *Advances in Nursing Science, 13*(4), 1–13.

National Center for Health Statistics. (1985). *National Health Interview Survey.* Vital and Health Statistics, Series 10, No. 150. DHHS Pub. No. (PHS) 85-1578. Washington, DC: U.S. Government Printing Office.

O'Leary, P. A., McGill, J. S., Jones, K. E., & Paul, P. B. (1990). Gerontological research: Is it useful for nursing practice? *Journal of Gerontological Nursing, 16*(5), 28–32.

Robinson, L. D. (1981). Gerontological nursing research. In I. M. Burnside (Ed.). Nursing and the aged (2nd ed.) (pp. 654–666). New York: McGraw-Hill.

Strumpf, N., & Evans, L. K. (1988). Physical restraint of the hospitalized elderly: Perceptions of patients and nurses. *Nursing Research, 37*(3), 132–136.

Strumpf, N. E., Evans, L. K., Wagner, J., & Patterson, J. (1992). Reducing physical restraints: Developing an educational program. *Journal of Gerontological Nursing, 18* (11), 21–27.

Strumpf, N., Evans, L., Williams, C., & Williams, T. F. (1992, April). Patterns of care in restraint-free facilities: Lessons from abroad. *Search, 14*(5).

U.S. Department of Commerce, Bureau of the Census. (1987). *An aging world.* International Population Reports Series P-95, No. 78. Washington, DC: U.S. Government Printing Office.

U.S. Department of Health & Human Services. (1988). *Urinary incontinence in adults.* National Institutes of Health Consensus Development Conference Statement (Vol. 7, No. 5). Washington, DC: U.S. Government Printing Office.

Waldo, D. R., Sonnefeld, S. T., McKusick, D. R., & Arnett, R. H. (1989, Summer). Health expenditures by age group, 1977 and 1987. *Health Care Financing Review, 10*(4), 111–120.

Wells, T. J., Brink, C. A., Diokno, A. C., Wolfe, R., & Gillis, G. L. (1991). Pelvic muscle exercise for stress urinary incontinence in elderly women. *Journal of the American Geriatric Society, 39,* 785–791.

Wolanin, M. O. (1983). Clinical geriatric nursing research. In *Annual Review of Nursing Research,* Volume 1, pp. 75–99.

3

Empirical Trial and Error: Learning from Practice

Joanne Rader

INTRODUCTION

Trial and error, or empirical learning, can be a useful approach to determining the care needs of persons with dementia. Empirical learning involves using experience and observation as the bases for developing knowledge to guide practice. It also implies making mistakes and learning from them. When I honored what my colleagues and I were experiencing and observing while caring for residents with dementia, I had some very positive and enlightening experiences. Each "knowing" led to another, culminating in my current work on decreasing the use of physical restraints. It is my hope that sharing my experiences of empirical learning will give others the courage and conviction to reflect on what they have learned and are learning through trial and error in clinical practice.

SERVE PROGRAM

In 1983, when I was a clinical specialist in mental health nursing in a nursing home, the staff came to me with a problem on one of our twenty-four-bed units. Four very mobile, wandering residents were admitted within one month. They were restless and disoriented; they attempted to leave frequently and became combative when they were prevented from leaving. The staff told me I had to "do something" because the wandering residents were becoming very disruptive. At that time, the approach to managing wandering behavior was to orient residents to the reality that the nursing home was now their home, to tell them not to leave, to physically prevent them from leaving, and, if all else failed, to tie them into the chair.

Having completed graduate school just 3 years before, I was pretty sure there was not a lot available in the literature to guide my interventions; however, I knew of one paper (Sawyer, 1983) that described a program in which wanderers were taken off the regular unit for a day of special activities in a separate room. It is important to remember that, at this time, special care units for persons with dementia existed in only a few isolated facilities. Reality orientation was the only "therapy" in the literature to guide practitioners caring for persons with dementia, and my experience with that had been negative.

I knew that, at our facility, we could not set up a separate space or all-day program for these residents. However, I realized that the staff and other residents needed some respite, just as the wanderers did. Based on my observations of dementing illnesses, I knew that individuals in this phase of dementia have a short attention span, are restless and easily distracted, have difficulty following directions, and do not do well in traditional group activities. In addition, they generally feel frustrated and unsuccessful in their daily living activities.

I designed a special program called SERVE, an acronym for self-esteem, relaxation, vitality, and exercise, (Schwab, Rader, & Doan, 1985). This program consisted of music, exercise, games, touch, and relaxation. We implemented it in a small group setting for an hour, three times a week. The primary goal of this program was to structure activities so that residents would be successful and encouraged by their involvement. Although the SERVE program was helpful—residents participated in the program, enjoyed it, and returned to the unit less restless—it did not stop all the wandering episodes.

VERBAL AND NONVERBAL COMMUNICATION STRATEGIES

The SERVE group became a learning laboratory for me; indeed, much of what I have discovered about behaviors and approaches to dementia came from this experience. For example, I learned to fine-tune my verbal communication skills. Mr. S. taught me that it is important to tell persons with dementia exactly what you want them to do, in concrete terms. During one session, I wanted him to throw the beach ball he held in his hands. He seemed not to know what to do with it, so I told him, "Keep the ball moving." He proceeded to rotate the ball in his hands. When I observed this, I altered my words and told him, "Throw the ball," which he did. This same gentle man would pull the fire alarms on the unit. When I read what the label on the alarm said, I realized that he was simply following the concrete part of the directions, "Pull," and was unable to comprehend the abstract part, "in case of fire," because of his dementia. From experiences like these, I developed a list of communication strategies and taught staff to be very concrete and specific when they gave directions to residents.

I also began to realize that when we prevented residents from leaving the building, we really did not know where they would go or what they would do if they were able to follow through with this desire.

So, on a cold, sunny, winter day, when Helen calmly told the nurse that it was time to go home now, that she had to help her sister with the garden, I was notified and I asked Helen's permission to accompany her. She said she really could see no need for me to waste my time. She knew the way very well, and I probably had more important things to do; but she agreed that I could go. I paced my walking with hers. I told the staff to send out a search party if we were not back in thirty minutes. Then I simply walked outside with Helen and tried to follow her lead using basic communication skills in addition to those I had learned through the SERVE program.

I found it easier to physically redirect and reroute her when I followed her lead by asking her questions about her sister and their garden. In a sense, I was following her agenda and bringing her sister to her through skillful communication. I tried to create the state of mind she was seeking in our relationship and interactions.

As we walked, I noticed that she was becoming uncertain and confused about what direction to go. I took this as an indication that she might be open to guidance if I could find a way to redirect her into the building without her having to admit she was confused or lost. It seemed very important that this resident *not* be confronted by her own confusion. People suffering from dementia need ways to save face, just as we do. So I commented that it was very cold outside and my legs were tired, and asked her if she was cold and tired. She said she was. I told her that I knew a place we could go to get warm and rested, and asked whether she would like to come along. She said she would. I counted on her distractibility and loss of short-term memory to help me redirect her, along with the concreteness of cold and fatigue as a motivator.

AGENDA BEHAVIOR

I accompanied other residents when they wandered, and I began to see common elements in behaviors related to wishing to leave the facility. First, people were asking to return to a time and place where they felt loved, needed, secure, safe, or in control. It wasn't the last apartment they had lived in with their spouse, but somewhere much further back in time. In fact, when I accompanied several residents and their spouses to the home they had left to come to the nursing home, they requested to go "home" in that environment also. I sensed that they were seeking not so much a geographic place as a state of mind. Our wanderings were not always without incident. I ended up in the same local bar on two separate occasions with different women, one of whom ordered drinks for the house!

These wandering residents were still cognitively intact enough to have some plan of action and some need appeared to be driving that plan of action. For example, one gentleman informed me that he needed to leave because he had to go mow the lawn. I interpreted his plan of action to reflect an underlying need to be busy and to be of service. I told him that I understood his need to mow the lawn, but right now I had a task that only he could help me with and asked if he would be willing to stay and assist me. I counted on his impaired memory and distractibility to again serve me well, if I could get him involved in an activity in the building that met his underlying need to be of service. In all of these examples, the residents' desire and will to leave only intensified if staff attempted to orient them to current reality and thwarted their physical efforts to leave.

These experiences related to exit-seeking wandering led me to the idea of agenda behavior (Rader, Doan, & Schwab, 1985), defined as the verbal and nonverbal planning and actions that cognitively impaired persons use in an effort to fulfill their social, emotional, and physical needs. The actions may or may not be related to current reality or to staff or family agendas. The primary cause of agenda behavior is thought to be the fear engendered by separation, both physical and cognitive, from the people and situations with which the person was previously most connected and comfortable. The agenda is undertaken to recapture those old satisfying situations, which formerly brought feelings of safety and belonging.

Although this concept has not been "scientifically" tested, its clinical usefulness continues to be demonstrated in my own practice, as well as in that of many other practitioners and educators who communicate its effectiveness to me through letters and comments.

COMPREHENSIVE APPROACH
TO WANDERING

I observed that when wandering behavior was managed by the common 3-step intervention of (1) reality orientation, (2) thwarting the agenda, and (3) physical and chemical restraints, many residents lost the ability to independently ambulate in as little as 2 weeks. A new, more comprehensive approach was needed. Based on our previous work on communication and the SERVE program, our facility decided that it was inappropriate to restrain residents for wandering behavior and implemented an alternative strategy that included: (1) problem identification, (2) preventive activities and programs, (3) appropriate verbal and nonverbal interactions, and (4) development of a staff mobilization plan in case staff were unable to locate a wandering resident (Rader, 1987). These four approaches could be implemented with minimal time and expense, and they effectively increased the safety of exit-seeking wanderers, without restricting their mobility. An important part of this strategy was working closely with families and explaining that risks are inherent in life and potentially dangerous behaviors, such as wandering away or falling, do not, and should not, cease to exist when someone enters a nursing home.

RESTRAINT REDUCTION

I am currently using empirical learning in decreasing the use of physical restraints for residents at risk of falling. In this area, health care practitioners have allowed fear of liability to drive practice. We have overestimated the benefits of physical restraints and underestimated the burdens. We have felt that we should prevent all falls and that we were at fault if we did not. We have treated each fall as if it were a potentially terminal event, although 95% of falls do not result in injury.

Changing and updating practice related to falls requires not only that we become familiar with current research and examine our outdated attitudes and biases, but also that we interpret our experiences and observations in light of new findings (Rader & Donius, 1991). For example, what should staff do when they have a disoriented resident recovering from hip replacement surgery who has fallen once, can't remember to ask for help, forgets to use her walker, and becomes verbally and physically aggressive when restraints are used or her mobility is restricted in any way? What my colleagues have learned to do is carefully assess why she fell and see if the cause can be corrected; assess the placement of furniture in her room so that the walker and objects can be used safely for support; assess her shoes and gait for ways to increase safety; and develop a system for alerting the staff when she stands so that they can quickly assist her. In addition, we have explained the risks of restraint use to the resident's daughter, to have her understand that her mother would be at risk of falling even if restraints were used. We have also explained that we have other ways to increase, although not ensure her mother's safety and that her mother has clearly indicated that she does not wish to be restrained. We observed that restraints create a tremendous physical and emotional burden for her.

This woman, in spite of two additional noninjury falls, is currently an independent but disoriented ambulator, seen frequently and happily asking for redirection to her "home" or room. Had we kept her "safe" by restraining her, she would not have returned to independent ambulation.

SUMMARY

To make this kind of dramatic shift in attitude and practice related to restraint use and falls requires that nurses fine-tune their observational and assessment skills, so they can learn from past experiences. Trial-and-error learning is most important when change in practice precedes much of the scientific work.

Long-term care nursing practice is not for sissies. It requires a great deal of courage to "allow" residents to fall. However, if each individual is thoughtfully assessed in light of what is learned from experience with other residents, it becomes easier and confidence builds.

It occurred to me several years ago that, somewhere along the way, I had become confident of my nursing abilities. I had spent many years feeling that I was incompetent because I didn't "know" enough, so this was a wonderful surprise. I realized I had a new definition of confidence that served me well. Confidence is knowing what you know, knowing what you don't know, and having the courage to admit to both.

REFERENCES

Rader, J. (1987). Comprehensive approach to problem wandering. *The Gerontologist, 27*(6), 756–760.

Rader, J., Doan, J., & Schwab, M. (1985, July/August). How to decrease wandering, a form of agenda behavior. *Geriatric Nursing, 6*(4), 196–199.

Rader, J., & Donius, M. (1991). Leveling off restraints. *Geriatric Nursing, 12*(2), 71–73.

Sawyer, J. (1983, November). *A management program for ambulatory institutionalized patients with Alzheimer's disease and related disorders.* Paper presented at the Annual Conference of the Gerontological Society, Boston.

Schwab, M., Rader, J., & Doan, J. (1985). SERVE: A management program for persons with Dementia. *Journal of Gerontological Nursing, 11*(5), 8–15.

4

No More Long Halls, No More Yellow Walls: Knowledge-Based Nursing Home Design

Janet Ikenn Fine

THE HIDDEN HEALTH CARE CRISIS

According to the Agency for Health Care Policy and Research (ACHPR), in a study titled *The Risk of Nursing Home Use in Later Life* (1990), more than 40% of all Americans 65 years of age or older will spend some portion of their remaining years in a nursing home. This stay will exceed 5 years for 1 out of every 5 individuals. For those who turned age 65 in 1990, future nursing home care is projected to cost $60 billion (ACHPR, 1991). Rising costs are not the only concern. The burgeoning numbers of older adults in the United States who require nursing home care will more than double by the year 2040. The stage is set for older adults to experience major difficulties in obtaining sufficient long-term care services in the near future. (See Figure 4.1.)

Despite the great expense and growing need, little scientific attention has been paid to the design, functionality, or efficacy of the nursing home as a therapeutic environment. In actuality, according to Rep. Edward Roybal (D-CA), departing chairman of the House Select Committee on Aging, less than 1% of the money spent on health care for the elderly is allocated to research (staff, 1992). As a major part of the health care delivery system for increasing numbers of older adults, the efficiency and

Figure 4.1
Age and the Need for Long-Term Care

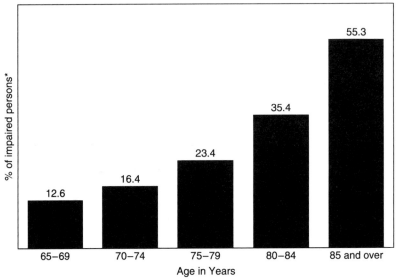

(*Percent with impaired abilities to conduct activities of daily living or to perform basic functions that support these activities.)

The Aged, Nursing Home Use and Nursing

- By 2040, the number of persons 65 and over will more than double, from 30 million to 67 million.
- By 2040, the number of persons over 85 will quadruple.
- Only 1% of persons aged 65–74 are in nursing homes; 22% of persons aged 85 and over are in nursing homes.

Source: Health Care Financing Administration, *Health Care Financing Review*, 1988 Annual Supplement. Reproduced with permission.

effectiveness of nursing home care warrants closer scrutiny—particularly because many legislators and their constituents may well have reason to doubt the cost-effectiveness of this type of health care environment.

Rooted in a medical model, both the organizational and the physical aspects of nursing homes remain far more suited to short-term stays by the acutely ill than to long-term residency by those with chronic conditions. Administrators, staff, residents, architects, and environmental designers are all increasingly aware of these limitations. Over the past fifteen years, a small but increasingly vocal number of researchers have undertaken studies documenting the problems of current long-term care environments (Calkins, 1990; Cohen & Weisman, 1991; Hiatt, 1992; Koncelik, 1976). These and other authors contend that more residential and therapeutic designs for nursing homes must be considered in future construction (Cohen & Day, 1991; Hiatt, 1980, 1981a, 1981b, 1982, 1984, 1987; Lawton, Fulcomer, & Kleban, 1984). To date, however, there have been only a very limited number of demonstration projects, severely handicapping researchers' ability to assess the efficacy of alternative approaches.

Such delay may have catastrophic consequences. The National Center for Health Statistics has postulated that meeting the demand for nursing home beds by the year 2025 will require building eight 100-bed nursing homes every week from now until that time. If the supply of nursing home beds is on such a compelling and impending collision course with demand, research concerning innovation, efficacy, and cost-effectiveness may well be crucial. How is it then that the current ineffective model has remained unchallenged?

Twenty-five years ago, nursing homes as we know them today were created as sociopolitical experiments spawned by new federal entitlement programs (Medicare and Medicaid). Unwittingly, architecture was based on the only inpatient care model known at the time, the hospital. In retrospect, nursing homes as we know them have really been a design experiment. This model may have been well-suited to the short-term, acutely ill person of an earlier era, but it certainly did not anticipate the significant differences in the needs of the long-term older adult of today. Nursing homes are no longer short-term "way stations" for older adults between acute care and mortuary care. Improved technological and medical advances have resulted in the need for people to cope longer with chronic illness than they ever have before. Such advances have also had significant impact on clients of the modern nursing home who, in the not-so-distant past, might not have survived a medical crisis and been given a hospital discharge. Now, admitted to nursing homes for extended care, they face uncertain futures and longer dependency than they ever anticipated.

Older adults have become increasingly disenchanted with technology that seems to prolong the length of their lives without thought to the quality. As harsher economic times prevail, the need for increasing numbers of women to join the labor force has compromised the ability of many families to provide long-term care for loved ones at home. Forced out of hospitals by prospective and capitate payment systems, increasing numbers of chronically ill older adults who have no other source of needed care are being discharged to nursing homes that were designed for short-term use by older adults of a bygone era and are ill-equipped to meet the needs of today's clientele.

A DEAF EAR AND A BLIND EYE

The emergence of this architectural crisis, this mismatch of form and function, could have been anticipated had we only listened to consumers. For years, they have pleaded, "Don't EVER put me in a nursing home!" Cries for construction and program reform have been systematically ignored because of short-sighted but compelling concerns about the escalating cost of long-term health care. Over the past decade, while academics and reformists have called for change, three major issues have all but eliminated the ability to research more cost-effective and efficient designs and equipment:

1. Moratoriums on nursing home construction in many states have been enacted to stem the proliferation of beds. Enactment of alternative programs to meet the increasing need for chronic illness care, however, has not kept pace. Simple limits on construction have merely meant cost shifting, not cost saving. In many instances, these legislative decisions have merely resulted in increasing the taxpayers' share of needlessly inflated health care.

2. Requirements for bureaucratic approval of Certificates of Need have included cost formulas that involve severely restrictive limits on spending per bed. Such formulas frequently have not been sufficiently indexed for inflation in construction or labor costs, nor have they recognized the value of incorporating modern workplace design to save costs over the full life cycle of the proposed structure.

3. Historic design codes have continued to be applied based on dogmatic rather than factual interpretations. Central nurses' stations, for example, might have had a purpose when the only way for a patient to attract the nurse's attention was to throw some object out into the hallway. Routine use of more sophisticated communication devices in modern times, however, still

has not resulted in the ability of providers to readily gain approval for designs that eliminate this central "command post." And so, the acute-care model has been perpetuated.

BREAKING THE STALEMATE

It is time to break the stalemate between controlling nursing home construction cost in the short term and preventing future escalation of long-term health care costs. As recently demonstrated by Alexian Village of Milwaukee, a lifecare retirement community, knowledge-based design may be an effective way to do just that. Continuing research now under way on this unique blend of structure and programming will attempt to validate explicit "design hypotheses." These hypotheses suggest that thoughtful design can enhance resident independence, improve staff efficiency, and result in improved quality of life for both.

Built in 1978, this facility's design of the former 61-bed nursing home section was typical of its time. Long, double-loaded corridors projected in a V-shape from a central nurses' station. Corridor lengths of 180 feet connected residents' rooms to centralized supply areas. Long walking distances and inconvenient or nonexistent supply storage made resident care duties needlessly time-consuming. Small rooms with side-by-side beds made provision of even the simplest nursing procedures difficult, and the promotion of resident independence was close to impossible. Privacy for staff and residents was nonexistent. Constantly changing duty assignments limited the staff's ability to learn residents' habits and accommodate familiar patterns of behavior.

Furnishings, while utilitarian, often fostered dependence and rarely resembled their residential counterparts. Large pieces of equipment and wheelchair-bound residents lined the corridors; both had no place else to go. Color choices and patterns—yellow painted walls, orange tiled floors, and small, nondistinct repeating-pattern fabrics—were combined with shadow-producing decorative light sconces on the walls. Such furnishings were perfectly acceptable for nursing home use at the time the structure was built. However, based on more current information about how physical changes in the aging eye and brain affect the sensory needs of elderly persons, the furnishings could not have been more poorly chosen. Lack of sound-reducing materials and equipment produced a never-ending cacophony of buzzers and beeps that contributed to sensory overload for residents as well as for staff and visitors. What should have been a peaceful and supportive environment more closely resembled a battlefront staging area with much of the same stress-producing hustle and bustle!

When the decision was made to build a replacement nursing home, staff and residents alike agreed that they did not want to reproduce their current architectural problems. Recuperated residents from the retirement community who had temporarily been nursing home patients in the past appreciated the quality of care they received but recognized the glaring inadequacies in the physical plant design. Both residents and staff knew that if they continued to do what had always been done before, they would undoubtedly end up with the same result. Fortified by a common belief that change was long overdue, multiple focus groups were convened among residents, caregivers, and experts in nursing home design to create a new vision. With no preexisting conditions, they began with the simple question: "If you could design the ideal nursing home, what would it look like?"

From this collaborative perspective, three design principles emerged:

1. Build a residence for older adults who need nursing care for their chronic illnesses but who do not want their entire lives to be centered around that care.

2. Create a facility that enables residents to maintain their independence instead of one that fosters dependence.

3. Design a structure that combines both centralized and decentralized operations in a way that promotes staff efficiency and effective delivery of resident services.

Unique features in structural design (including one of the earliest constructions of an L-shaped semiprivate room), interior furnishings, and changes in service delivery were carefully intertwined to facilitate desired behavioral and attitudinal outcomes on the part of both residents and staff. With a shared vision for the future, strategic planning to gain the necessary regulatory acceptance began.

STRATEGY FOR SUCCESS

Knowing that both the design and its anticipated construction cost would be controversial, the planners notified the Secretary of the State Division of Health and Human Services (DHHS) that an unusual Certificate of Need was being submitted. The facility argued that this design could be a successful field test and wrote the design with the expectation that a legal challenge would most likely result. A detailed rationale for each controversial area was included within the application. Prior to submitting the Certificate of Need, the facility held meetings with regulators and department officials to explain why it felt compelled to challenge what had always been accepted in the past. Privately, many of those contacted believed in the need for change. Publicly, however, they vocalized a political need to enforce historically accepted interpretations and limitations of current statutes. Noting this discrepancy, the facility's strategy became a deliberate campaign of politics and persistence, designed to increase the leverage of those very private viewpoints.

Residents of the retirement community were a vital element of this strategy. Armed with details supplied by administrators, they began a systematic letter-writing campaign to convince the regulators of the need to approve the new nursing home model. Enlisting the aid of family members and friends, they wrote over 100 letters to the Governor, the DHSS Secretary, legislators, and influential friends, explaining the need to create a new model. They cited personal examples to help illustrate their needs and concerns, suggesting that governmental officials would do well to consider changes that might benefit their own later years.

Resistance to the change was formidable. Regardless of the potential benefits, the possibility of future demands on an already strained budget still seemed daunting to those whose public posture required restraint. Even under mounting pressure, their abandonment of a historically conservative approach for an uncertain and seemingly more expensive future seemed dubious.

Simultaneous with the approach taken by the residents, the facility decided to modify its application strategy by applying an allocation methodology to the required cost formula. A nursing home that was part of a larger retirement community, they argued, was unique. Exterior design needed to coordinate with connecting buildings already existing on the campus. Portions of certain areas would be used by residents of the retirement community and should, therefore, not be included in the formula. Common use of kitchens, utilities, and other support systems dictated proportionate allocation of construction expense. In all, 60% of shared space (representing 23% of the total building) was reallocated to the retirement community; overall costs were decreased by 30%. Additional supporting documentation requested by the state required substantial amounts of unanticipated consultation, preparation, and expense. Would this be an acceptable strategy to permit public approval without compromising existing regulations?

Disappointingly, the allocation methodology was at first denied. Then, at the "eleventh hour," an emergency rule was unexpectedly promulgated by the Governor and passed by the legislature to increase the existing cost formula by more than 15% per bed. The facility's proposal was quickly approved. Construction plans, which had continued to be formulated during the uncertainty of the long bureaucratic struggle, were immediately implemented. Fifteen months later, in August 1991, the entire population of the existing nursing home relocated to their new 87-bed residence. At a construction cost of over $5 million, this 70,600-square-foot, state-of-the-art, cluster model included the principles first envisioned by the focus groups of residents, staff, and consultants three years earlier.

SELECTION OF THE CLUSTER MODEL

While strategies were being developed to gain state approval for construction, architectural building design had proceeded. Administrators and architects (Ellerbe Becket, MN; Holland and Steed, IL) were unified in their determination to base as many design decisions as possible on the three principles elicited from focus group discussions: residential atmosphere, independence promotion, and staff efficiency. Dr. Lorraine Hiatt, nationally recognized for her work in environmental design for older adults and an early consultant on the project, suggested that a "cluster model" might best be able to capture these principles. This model was nontraditional in its approach. It used smaller, more residential-sized units, decentralized support areas for staff efficiency, and emphasized the spatial relationships between private and social areas. Prior to consideration of the cluster model, other designs had merited serious consideration because of the project's geographical location and unusual topography. Once introduced, however, the cluster design was quickly selected because of its unique ability to help achieve the project's design objectives. Tables 4.1 and 4.2 outline the key benefits of the cluster design.

CLUSTER DEVELOPMENT

Development of the cluster itself was sequentially driven. A good deal of time had been devoted earlier to selecting the ideal resident assignment

Table 4.1
Benefits of Cluster Design in Resident Staff Interactions

For Staff	For Residents
Shorter walking distances	Quicker staff response
More efficient care	More positive relationships with caregivers
Proximity to residents; more visibility	More one-to-one time
Ability to simultaneously assist multiple residents	More rehabilitation time
Facilitation of learning residents' routines	Enhanced independence
Increased job satisfaction	More homelike appearance and atmosphere
Less dependence of residents on staff	More staff familiarity with individual needs
	Increased security (staff nearer, more visible)

Table 4.2
Benefits of Cluster Design in Common Areas

For Staff	For Residents
Ease of coaching rehabilitation	Improved quality of life
Clerical area for nursing assistants	Greater variety of choices
Living rooms, to provide social interactions with residents	Ability to explore
Variety, making resident satisfaction easier to achieve	Ease of seeing and hearing
Off-unit recreational events provide for break in routine	Living rooms designed to promote socialization
Unipurpose areas, to facilitate advance preparation	Options for privacy
Appropriate staff conference areas	Minimal depersonalization
	Promotion of self-esteem
	Familiar, family-sized dining groups
	Multiple visiting areas
	Unipurpose rooms, to minimize confusion

size and realizing the benefits listed in Table 4.3. Although resident demands on staff time were fairly cyclical, the sustained peak of activity routinely occurring during the first half of the second shift required special attention to efficiency and flexibility at this time. Consequently, an assignment size of 10 residents per nursing assistant on this shift served as the basis for determining the capacity of each cluster. Cluster size, in turn, was the basic element that drove exterior building design. Cluster length was kept to 80 feet and a "jog" in the corridor was created to minimize the long-tunnel effect typically seen in nursing homes and hotels. To accommodate resident preferences, 4 clusters, with 4 private and 3 semiprivate rooms in each, were arranged around a central service core on two separate residential floors. Clusters were further enhanced to include small living rooms, kitchenettes, accessible shower rooms, and clean and soiled linen storage areas. A bathroom model was "mocked-up" in the existing community center so that alternative placement of fixtures and doorways could be tested by residents in wheelchairs. Eventually, efficient bathrooms were designed on 7-foot centers and furnished with swing-away grab bars, low recessed medicine chests for resident use, and linen closets for staff use. Table 4.4 lists all the features of the design.

Bedroom furnishings were designed and selected to be residential in character while enhancing resident independence. Each room had been designed with large, low, individual windows equipped with wood-appearing formica ledges to accommodate plants. Wall-mounted overbed lighting was discarded in favor of color-coordinated, brass-accented table lamps designed for use by the physically and mentally challenged. Durably manufactured with nightlights and additional electrical outlets

Table 4.3
Benefits of Cluster Design in
Staffing Patterns

Higher-quality assessments and evaluation of care
Responsiveness to changes in census or acuity
Support of unit-based vs. shift-based management
More efficient supervision by licensed staff
Support of case management
Support of practice partnerships
Support of flexible shifts
Defined areas of accountability
Staff training directed to specific resident types

Table 4.4
Unique Features of the Resident Bathroom

Sufficient floor space to turn/angle wheelchair independently

Accordion door, to allow wide access for independent wheelchair use or multiple staff assist

Swing-away grab bar, to maximize floor space for 1- or 2-person transfer and assist

Toilet height that enables lateral transfers

Counter and mirror height appropriate for seated resident

Vanity counter reinforced for use as standing support

Non-slip flooring even when wet

Individual linen closets for staff supplies

Individual medicine chests for residents' supplies

Low placement of tissue holder, towel bars, and medicine chests to facilitate accessibility by seated residents

included in their weighted bases, these lamps were an immediately visible symbol that connoted "residence" instead of "health care facility." Closets were abandoned as too costly to include the sprinklers required by the building code and too inefficient and inaccessible for most residents to use. In their place, the staff designed a customized wardrobe, easily accessed, with movable rods and shelving that could be individually configured to meet each resident's needs. Individual air temperature and fan controls were installed in each room to promote comfort, autonomy, and individual choice. Semiprivate and private rooms alike were sized with 180 feet of living space per person, encouraging wheelchair users to independently access their furniture, windows, and beds. To further promote privacy, architect Dale Tremain's new L-shaped design for semiprivate rooms prevented direct lines of sight between the roommates' beds. A complete listing of the advantages offered by this design is given in Table 4.5.

INTERIOR DESIGN

Staff members were also instrumental in designing efficient interior spaces and testing possible furnishings and equipment. As former participants in focus groups and in the long campaign for design approval, they

Table 4.5
Unique Features of the L-Shaped
Semiprivate Room

Privacy for each resident

Defined personal territory

No direct sight line between beds

Individual windows and furniture

Access to personal areas without entering roommate's space
(i.e., closet, bathroom, etc.)

Ample space to provide seating for visitors

were already familiar with the identified design principles. Close communication between architects and staff helped to determine the optimum blend of decentralized and centralized work areas. (See Table 4.6.) They reasoned that the work of nursing assistants should be supported by decentralizing linen and hygiene supplies, but they believed that items requiring frequent monitoring or more control should be centrally located. Dining, medication, and treatment rooms, it was agreed, should still remain centralized. Electrical outlets formerly were hidden behind the bed just above the baseboard, an inconvenient location that frequently caused wall damage and muscle strain for staff trying to reach them. Now, they were placed beside the bed and were raised twenty-four inches from the

Table 4.6
Benefits of Cluster Design in
Supplies/Linens/Equipment

For Staff	For Residents
Supplies immediately available	No carts in halls
More rapid disposal of soiled items	More usable living area
	Less clutter
Hygiene items and equipment separated for each resident	Less waiting time
	Decreased chance of odor
Efficient restocking	Showers nearer rooms
More frequent rotation of supplies, to reduce wear and cost	Easier, safer independent movement
	Staff supplies not mixed with personal belongings

floor for easier access. To minimize resident confusion and maximize staff efficiency, dining rooms were designed to have one purpose (dining). In older designs, they had continually changed from meals to games to chapel to crafts. The color and seating in the dining rooms were deliberately designed to look and feel different from any other area in the facility so that residents would more easily associate the room with the dining experience.

The nursing station was carefully planned to accommodate staff needs while not violating the design's concern for maintaining a residential environment. From the regulatory point of view, this was one of the most controversial elements of the design. Conventional wisdom argued for locating the nursing station in the middle of the building, to permit unimpeded views down corridors, but a more enlightened nursing perspective found this reasoning to be faulty. How could resident dignity and self-esteem be enhanced without supporting the resident's right to privacy? Prevailing design code interpretations were based on a real concern for resident safety. A thorough review of historical incident report logs, however, showed that most resident incidents occurred in bedrooms and bathrooms, neither of which were visible from a central nursing station. Larger, more well-designed bedrooms and bathrooms were the key to promoting resident safety, not increased corridor surveillance. If a residential atmosphere was aesthetically desirable from a psychosocial perspective, the whole idea of a central command post had to be abandoned. Regardless of recent changes in federal nursing home requirements, which emphasized resident autonomy and more homelike environments,* regulators did not easily give up the tradition of a central nursing station. Nurses were equally determined that the design must respect resident privacy and that their main work area should be quietly recessed away from residential clusters and efficiently equipped to meet their needs. A last-minute compromise was reached: a small desk was located in the center of each cluster, to serve as a "substation" where nursing assistants could unobtrusively observe resident activities while they worked.

Finally, great care was taken to reduce the sensory overload so apparent in the former building's design. A nurse call-signal system was chosen that would accommodate two-way voice communication with the traditional audible signal but permit the use of nonaudible visual signals as

---

* Omnibus Budget Reconciliation Act (OBRA), Subtitle C, Nursing Home Reform, P.L. 100-203 (1987; effective 1990). Text available from U.S. Government Printing Office, Washington, DC.

well. Rather than using audible alarms to alert staff to danger, the electronic wander control system selected had the ability to deny door access by means of magnetic locks temporarily and noiselessly triggered when a wanderer entered the zone. To further support the objective of creating a peaceful, residential environment, a unique no-pile carpet-like flooring was selected for its sound-absorbing property as well as its cleanability. Use of a random, unbordered carpet design throughout the clusters minimized visual distortion and the typical perception of thresholds at the entrance to each room, where room and corridor patterns differ. Finally, the design itself was complemented by wall treatments and fabrics appropriate for the user with true non-yellowing colors and large, distinct patterns clearly defining the backgrounds from the foregrounds. Color combinations and artwork were also varied in each cluster to facilitate way finding.

MOVING PARTNERSHIPS

The move was planned as deliberately as the building's design. A significant amount of relocation research had suggested that the most serious consequences occurred when older adults were not included in the planning process (Amenta, Weiner, & Amenta, 1984; Borup, Gallego, & Heffernan, 1980; Burnette, 1986; Mirotznik & Ruskin, 1984, 1985; Moos, David, Lemke, & Postle, 1984; Pino, Rosica, & Carter, 1978; Rosswurm, 1983; Thomasma, Yeaworth, & McCabe, 1990; Young, 1990). To mitigate the possibility of creating unanticipated negative effects even when the move itself was beneficial, "moving partnerships" were deliberately formed. Each of the frail, elderly residents and his or her family were partnered by a specially trained, staff member 6 months before the move. Briefing sessions held periodically for these staff members kept them current with design decisions, anticipated changes, and potential problems. Similar family meetings were held. Residents who historically had difficulty with change were referred to specialists for additional assistance. Moving partners, serving as information resources and friends, were to be instrumental in preparing residents and their families for the changes that were to come.

Week by week, moving partners carefully structured activities designed to help residents stay focused on the move ahead and remain active as participants in the planning process. Based on research done at the University of Wisconsin (Hunt, 1984; Hunt & Gunter-Hunt, 1983), a portable model of the new building was constructed with movable clusters and removable ceilings so it could be used to help familiarize residents with the relationship between pathways and locations where they would live. Using the model, routes from the clusters to the dining room, nursing station, and TV lounges could be demonstrated when talking about their new home. Enlarged sections of blueprints and construction-in-progress photographs were hung in the hallways of the existing structure as daily reminders of the move ahead. A "count-down calendar" placed at the door to the dining room announced the remaining days until the move would occur. Residents were encouraged to choose their own room locations and decide how their personal belongings and furnishings would be arranged. Some residents were eager for the private rooms that would now be available to them. Others, however, thought they would be lonely after having lived with a roommate for so long and chose semi-private accommodations. "What would she do without me?" one woman asked. Watching over a roommate gave purpose to her life. Miraculously, almost everyone's choices were accommodated by the new design. Together, moving partners and residents packed up personal possessions and moved them through the connecting link into the new building. Over the many months of preparation, bonds of trust and friendly relationships had developed serendipitously between residents and their moving partners. On moving day and during the weeks that followed, these new "friends" took special care to help their residents become acclimated to their new surroundings. With careful planning, what could have been a most difficult event transformed observers into participants and became a tangible source of satisfaction and pride.

COMBINING FORM AND FUNCTION

Much debate has centered around the creation of special dementia units versus the benefits of having demented residents reside alongside those more cognitively intact. Because of its historical experience, this facility chose to create distinctly separate units. As a lifecare facility, the nursing home had consistently experienced a high number of short-term recuperative admissions. During their temporary stay, recuperating residents had frequently expressed their discomfort at living with the constantly disruptive behaviors of their now cognitively impaired relatives and neighbors. The rapid pace of temporary admissions and discharges also compromised the demented resident's clinical need for environmental consistency.

The new building design, therefore, intentionally separated residents. Those with significant cognitive impairments were on a different floor from those whose primary needs were more physical. Many meetings were held to discuss the differences in nursing staff expectations and the required training for each of the two floors. Continuing a long-standing commitment to staff (as well as to resident) empowerment, staff members were encouraged to choose the particular type of residents with whom they wished to work.

Programs were restructured to complement the new philosophy and design. If the individuality and needs of each resident were to be the focus of care delivery, relationships between residents and staff needed to be deliberate and constant. Practice partnerships were envisioned between nurses and nursing assistants on each floor, curtailing the traditional movement of staff from assignment to assignment. Non-nursing duties such as serving trays and distributing linen were reassigned to other departments which prioritized nursing time for resident assistance.

Pursuing a belief that program and building should be integrated, the work of support departments was reevaluated, to scrutinize how and when work was accomplished. Interior design was used as a means to support the work: traffic patterns and supply storage were designed to be more efficient. Service delivery became seen as a way to enable resident autonomy, dignity, and choice, and non-nursing staff considered what changes they needed to make. Departments such as Housekeeping, Dining Services, and Recreational Therapy revised staffing patterns and work routines to accommodate more resident choices. For example, using a residential service model, the Dining Services Department altered its staffing patterns to permit restaurant-style instead of tray-line service. Clerical and office work changes were also required by the building's new structure. Because of the new structural design and placement of the nursing station, the unit secretary's desk now became the reception area for each of the residential floors. Administrative offices, located on the ground floor, were furnished to support more efficient work flow and communication patterns. Rehabilitative and recreational therapies were purposely located on this floor, away from the clusters, to provide a complete change of atmosphere for a resident who attended and to offer cluster staff a break from that resident's care. Perhaps the most dramatic of all departmental restructuring occurred in the Recreational Therapy Department. Once centralized in a single small room, the activities of this department were fundamentally changed to provide specialized programming in two residential TV lounges and 8 cluster living rooms; a large, central community center and kitchen; and a specialized arts and crafts room.

SHARED VISION, SHARED GOALS

Residents and staff have occupied their new building for about 1½ years. Fortunately, future research possibilities were envisioned and data were gathered prior to the move, for comparative use in ongoing studies in the new structure. (The former nursing home has since been converted to a residential assisted living center.) Two distinct research studies are currently proceeding under the auspices of the University of Wisconsin. The first project, conducted by an experienced nurse researcher and clinician, is looking at the nursing management of resident health problems over time. The second project, under the direction of the University of Wisconsin School of Architecture and Urban Planning, is being conducted by graduate students studying resident use of social and living spaces. Both of these studies will compare data gathered in the old building with data gathered in the new one. Results are anticipated in late 1993. A recently completed, noncomparative third study was conducted by the facility Administrator. Developed as a postoccupancy evaluation, its focus was to ascertain whether the anticipated outcomes of critical design decisions in twenty-seven different areas would be validated by staff experience. The fifty-nine multidisciplinary respondents (50% return rate) were overwhelmingly positive about improvements realized by the architecture and furnishings. Only 6% of the responses to over three hundred questions indicated that the desired objective had not occurred.

Perhaps related to efforts of the moving partners to keep residents fully involved in the planning process, anticipated increases in morbidity and mortality did not occur. Although the average age of the sixty relocated residents was 87, the death rate for this group during the first 12 months following occupancy was actually 15% less than that of the two prior years. Clinical improvements have also been recognized after an initial adjustment period. Initially, behavior problems in the cognitively impaired resident population did dramatically increase. Confused residents, now separated from the general population, predictably had more difficulty in orienting to their new environment and relating to one another. Over 6–9 months' time, however, as residents became more familiar with their new surroundings and staff increased their skills, these problems not only subsided but became less troublesome than in the former facility. Now, over a year later, the atmosphere in the clusters where these residents live is consistently calm and generally harmonious. As in the former nursing home, restraining devices are not routinely used and residents are free to roam about.

The number of resident falls, always a concern, has shown some interesting changes. After a brief initial period of increased falls, the total percentage of incidents involving falls during 1992 remained essentially the same as in 1990, the year prior to the move. Falls in resident bathrooms have decreased by 10%, as might have been predicted by the improvements designed to make them safer. Falls in the hallways, a major concern when debating the elimination of a central nursing station, decreased by 2%. Is the new building safer for residents? Remarkably, significant injuries have decreased by 50% from the prior year, resulting in corresponding reductions in the number of residents transferred to an emergency room or admitted to a hospital following an incident.

Nurses notice that residents sleep better, although there has been an ongoing campaign to minimize the use of psychotropic medications. Mealtimes are calmer as well, with less disruptive behavior and less straying away from the table. Residents eat better and socialize more during their meals. The ongoing efforts of staff members to reduce incontinence have at last resulted in a 16% improvement. An improved building design was not singularly responsible for this achievement. Efforts that had been under way for 2 years, however, are now fully supported by the convenience of accessible bathrooms and familiar staff who are more fully aware of their residents' daily needs.

The change in atmosphere is apparent upon entering the lobby, where soothing colors and recessed lighting complement several comfortable groupings of living room furniture, encouraging social conversation. This same ambiance is mirrored by the clusters themselves, on the upper floors. Gone are the harsh lights and raucous noises often associated with traditional nursing homes. Gone, too, are the halls lined with vacantly staring wheelchair-bound residents. Instead, the scene resembles what you would expect to see in any residential apartment building for older adults. Some people are socializing together, others are attending various activities and therapies, still others pursue individual interests in their rooms. Even in the clusters reserved for residents with cognitive impairments, along with the wandering and the rummaging and the pacing, there is still an air of peace. Rooms are decorated with treasured pieces of furniture and mementos. Family members and friends visit often and frequently remark that they are more comfortable in the new environment.

Residents are thrilled with their improved ability to maintain independence and seem delighted with their newfound privacy and dignity. As one resident summarized, "The nicest thing is that now I have choices again!" Staff members, over a year later, still take every opportunity to express unsolicited praise for the new nursing home. Definitive results have not yet materialized from the ongoing clinical research studies, but many of the immediate goals of staff and residents have already been realized.

IMPLICATIONS FOR THE FUTURE

These improvements, it is hoped, will provide continued impetus for dedicated gerontologists to continue educating the public about the need for environmental design changes in nursing homes. But this alone will not change prevailing attitudes toward spending sufficient dollars to enable frail, older adults to have dignity and independence. Research must continue to explore whether long-term savings can truly be realized by knowledge-based nursing home design. Observed results at this facility suggest that this may be so.

Administrative costs associated with staff recruitment have benefited from changes in building design. Even in the midst of a nursing shortage, over 50 experienced nurses applied for the half-dozen new positions required by the increased bed capacity of the new facility. Voluntary nursing staff turnover, though consistently low in this facility, decreased by an additional 13% in the first full year following construction. Of particular note is that the four clusters for cognitively impaired residents have had only one staff member terminate voluntarily (due to family problems). In 1991, the Wisconsin Association of Homes and Services for the Aging reported that turnover costs long-term care facilities $1,550 per person, and that annual savings of over $80,000 could be realized if a facility could prevent the turnover of just one person per week. Based on these figures, an estimated $18,600 was saved from decreased turnover alone, in the new building's first year. With every expectation that the new building will last at least 40 years, a design that minimizes the cost of staff recruitment and retention could easily result in considerable savings.

The cost of nursing home care may be reduced by thoughtful design in other ways as well. If incontinence and other dependencies commonly (and wrongly) associated with aging and accepted as inevitable can be reduced by efficient nursing home design and coordinated clinical programs, then there is promise that the expense of labor-intensive nursing services can be reduced. If older adults with complex medical needs are aware that they can live in environments that are residential and dignified while still receiving the skilled care that they need, the fear and guilt associated with accepting necessary nursing home care can be minimized. Earlier intervention and rehabilitation may someday reduce the federal share of nursing home costs, but knowledge-based design in this facility has already been shown to improve resident life quality and staff satisfaction. It is hoped that the results of research on this innovative new structure will continue to influence improvements in nursing home design far into the future.

REFERENCES

Agency for Health Care Policy and Research. (1990). The risk of nursing home use in later life. *Medical Care, 28*(10), 952–962.

Agency for Health Care Policy and Research. (1991). Lifetime use of nursing home care. *New England Journal of Medicine, 324*, 595–600.

Amenta, M., Weiner, A., & Amenta, D. (1984). Successful relocation of elderly residents. *Geriatric Nursing, 5*(6), 356–360.

Borup, J., Gallego, D., & Heffernan, P. (1980). Relocation: Its effect on health, functioning, and mortality. *The Gerontologist, 20*(4), 468–479.

Burnette, K. (1986). Relocation and the elderly: Changing perspectives. *Journal of Gerontological Nursing, 12*(10), 6–11.

Calkins, M. (1990). *Design for dementia: Planning environments for the elderly and the confused.* Owings Mills, MD: National Health Publishing.

Cohen, U., & Day, K. (1991). *Contemporary designs for people with dementia.* Monograph Series: Institute of Aging and Environment. Milwaukee, WI: Publications in Architecture and Urban Planning (Report 91-4).

Cohen, U., & Weisman, J. (1991). *Holding on to home.* Baltimore, MD: Johns Hopkins University Press.

Health Care Financing Administration. (1988). *Health Care Financing Review,* Annual Supplement. Washington, DC: U.S. Government Printing Office.

Hiatt, L. (1980). Is poor light dimming the sight of nursing home patients? *Nursing Homes, 29*(5), 32–41.

Hiatt, L. (1981a). Color and use of color in environments for older people. *Nursing Homes, 30*(3), 18–22.

Hiatt, L. (1981b). Designing therapeutic dining. *Nursing Homes, 30*(2), 33–39.

Hiatt, L. (1982). The environment as a participant in health care. *Journal of Long Term Care Administration, 10*(1), 1–17.

Hiatt, L. (1984). Conveying the substance of images: Interior design in long-term care. *Contemporary Administrator, 4*, 17–19, 55.

Hiatt, L. (1987). Environmental design and mentally impaired older people. In H. Altman (Ed.), *Alzheimer's disease: Problems, prospects and perspectives.* New York: Plenum Press.

Hiatt, L. (1992). *Nursing home renovation: Design for reform.* Boston: Butterworth.

Hunt, M. (1984). Environmental learning without being there. *Environment and Behavior, 16*(3), 307–334.

Hunt, M., & Gunter-Hunt, G. (1983). Simulated site visits in the relocation of older people. *Health and Social Work, 8*, 5–14.

Koncelik, J. (1976). *Designing the open nursing home.* Stroudsburg, PA: Dowden, Hutchinson & Ross.

Lawton, P., Fulcomer, M., & Kleban, M. (1984). Architecture for the mentally impaired elderly. *Environment and Behavior, 16*(6), 730–757.

Mirotznik, J., & Ruskin, A. P. (1984). Interinstitutional relocation and its effects on health. *The Gerontologist, 24*(3), 286–291.

Mirotznik, J., & Ruskin, A. P. (1985). Interinstitutional relocation and the elderly. *The Journal of Long Term Care Administration, 13*(4), 127–131.

Moos, R., David, T., Lemke, S., & Postle, E. (1984). Coping with an intrainstitutional relocation: Changes in resident and staff behavior patterns. *The Gerontologist, 24*(5), 495–502.

Pino, C., Rosica, L., & Carter, T. (1978). The differential effects of relocation on nursing home patients. *The Gerontologist, 18*(2), 167–172.

Rosswurm, M. (1983). Relocation and the elderly. *Journal of Gerontological Nursing, 9*(12), 632–637.

Staff. (1992). More dollars needed for aging research: Testimony. *McKnight's Long Term News, 13*(5), 39.

Thomasma, M., Yeaworth, R., & McCabe, B. (1990). Moving day: Relocation and anxiety in institutionalized elderly. *Journal of Gerontological Nursing, 16*(7), 19–24.

Wisconsin Association of Homes and Services for the Aging (1991). News briefs. *The Communicator, 22*(1), 18.

Young, H. (1990). The transition of relocation to a nursing home. *Holistic Nursing Practice, 4*(3), 74–83.

5

Ways of Caring: Acute Care for Older Adults Without Restraints

Lois K. Evans

Many aspects of the acute-care hospital experience are harmful to the health and well-being of the older patient, particularly if the person is frail. A strange environment, without orienting cues or homelike features; multitudes of stranger caregivers, together with isolation from family and the familiar; noises, routines, and other stimuli that require adaptation and coping at a time when energy is best spent in recovery; and diagnostic and treatment regimens with a range of likely side effects make even an elective or "routine" hospital stay somewhat risky for the older adult. Current research confirms that older patients are at high risk of developing iatrogenic complications during a hospital stay (Stone, 1991). Among the most common is delirium, or acute confusional state, often the result of adverse drug reactions or physiologic changes accompanying illness or treatment. Immobilization results in development of pressure sores, nosocomial infections, muscle weakness, risk of falling, and decline in physical and mental function, including limitations in activities of daily living, difficulty eating, and incontinence. Complications from diagnostic and therapeutic measures are common. Patient behaviors, including confusion, agitation, sliding out of chair, climbing out of bed unassisted, and self-removal of an irritating intravenous line or feeding tube, result in nonconsensual treatment with physical restraint or psychoactive drugs, each with its own sequelae.

Since the birth of modern nursing, one function has been clear: "And what nursing has to do . . . is to put the patient in the best condition for nature to act upon him" (Nightingale, 1859, p. 75). Yet the condition "best" for the hospitalized older patient has been forgotten, or perhaps misunderstood. Tappen and Beckerman (1992) described families' complaints about nursing's failure to provide for some of the basic human needs that their hospitalized older relatives were unable to manage alone: maintenance of adequate nutrition and hydration, preservation of circulation and skin integrity, and protection against further harm. Respect for the individual's privacy and dignity and individualized, humanistic care were also perceived as lacking; relatives expressed many concerns regarding the physical restraint of their elder. Achieving Nightingale's goal will require a subtle but profoundly different way of perceiving and providing care to the hospitalized elderly, one that does not include the routine use of physical restraints.

HISTORY AND CURRENT STATUS OF
THE PRACTICE OF RESTRAINT

A physical restraint is defined as a device placed on or near the person's body that limits freedom of voluntary movement or free access to one's own body (Evans & Strumpf, 1989). Examples in common use today include vest, limb, waist, and pelvic restraints, and chairs with fixed tray tables. The nursing literature is rife with euphemisms—postural support, soft tie, jacket, safety belt, and so forth—that appear to make it easier to avoid acknowledgment of the actual purpose for the devices. Restraints have a long history of use for controlling dangerous behavior in the mentally ill, but their imbeddedness in practice with elders in acute and long-term care is more recent (Strumpf & Tomes, 1993). In fact, early nursing and all subsequent gerontologic nursing texts have cautioned against restraint of delirious patients because "it only makes them worse" (Weeks, 1885, p. 302); nevertheless, the literature increasingly provided guidelines for restraint use, and even instructions for constructing the devices, until they became commercially available in 1937. By the late 1980s, restraint use was a very common practice, particularly for "protection" of frail elders against fall risk, treatment interference, or disturbing behavior. Reportedly, 41% of nursing home residents, 22% of older acute hospital patients, and 34% of hospital-based rehabilitation unit patients were restrained on a regular basis (Strumpf & Evans, 1992).

The restrained tend to be sick and frail, having in common cognitive impairment, physical dependency, risk of falling, treatment devices in place, high illness severity index, and/or disruptive behavior (Evans & Strumpf, 1989). In the hospital, restrained elders, when compared with nonrestrained elders, have higher mortality rates, more adverse events (new pressure sores, nosocomial infections, complications, falls), a longer length of stay, and greater likelihood of discharge to a nursing home (Lofgren, McPherson, Granieri, Myllenbeck, & Sprafka, 1989); restraints do not protect from falls, and the restrained who fall have a greater risk of serious injury (Tinetti, Liu, & Ginter, 1992). Thus, the most frail are restrained, and restraint contributes to the development of additional frailty.

The following myths, now refuted by research, have encouraged continuation of the practice in spite of increasing evidence against it: That older patients are at greater risk of serious injury, that they need the protection that can best be afforded by physical restraint, that not restraining will result in legal liability, that being restrained has no emotional effect on older patients, that limited staffing requires restraint use, and that there are no other alternatives (Evans & Strumpf, 1990). Recent professional and public awareness of the hazards of restraint; changes in ethical and legal climates toward individual choice; recognition that restraints do not ensure safety; and rights advocacy resulting in nursing home reform legislation (OBRA, 1987)* requiring curtailment of physical restraint, have resulted in a significant reduction in restraint use in nursing homes. Two recent events are likely to have a similar impact in the acute-care setting. Because of increasing reports of injuries and deaths resulting from restraint use and misuse (Miles & Irvine, 1992), the Food and Drug Administration recently released safety alerts spelling out the known hazards associated with physical restraints, and proposed regulatory changes to enhance product labeling and user education (Weick, 1992). In 1991, the Joint Commission on Accreditation of Healthcare Organizations (JCAHO, 1991) disseminated changes in guidelines regarding the use of restraints, acknowledging the significant patient rights and risk issues involved. Experience in reducing restraints in long-term (Blakeslee, Goldman, Papougenis, & Torell, 1991; Evans & Strumpf, 1992) and acute-care settings (English, 1989; Mitchell-Pedersen, Fingerote, Powell, & Edmund, 1989) suggest that certain

---

* Omnibus Budget Reconciliation Act (OBRA), Subtitle C, Nursing Home Reform, P.L. 100-203 (1987; effective 1990). Text available from U.S. Government Printing Office.

factors are imperative for lasting change: administrative commitment and support, a philosophical shift in the paradigm of care for the older adult, careful policy development, interdisciplinary collaboration, and staff training to facilitate more appropriate response to the difficult behavior so often resulting in restraint.

REFRAMING AND RESPONDING
TO DIFFICULT BEHAVIOR

Behavior that interferes with the smooth delivery of care, is "noncompliant" with health care recommendations or routines, and/or causes distress to caregivers and others in the environment is often labeled "difficult." More often identified by the caregiver than by the one receiving care, "difficult behavior" can occur in any setting. Medical and psychiatric disorders, together with their concomitant treatment, may actually predispose patients to display such "difficult behaviors" as unsafe mobility, interference with medical treatment, or other disruptive/disturbing behaviors. Thus, older adults in hospitals and nursing homes are likely to display behaviors judged to be "difficult" or "disturbing," because of the high prevalence of delirium, dementia, and depression among medically ill elders.

One approach to changing practice is to change nurses' belief systems through education. Once nurses understand that restriction in movement by restraint generally results in poorer quality of care, development of more effective responses can be achieved. The essence of restraint reduction or elimination is change in practice with regard to "difficult" behavior. Required is a major paradigm shift—from dehumanizing, task- and control-oriented care to person-centered care that is more attuned to individual needs. "Making sense of behavior" is a fundamental component of individualized care (Evans, Strumpf, & Williams, 1992; Strumpf, Evans, Wagner, & Patterson, 1992). It is important to recall that all behavior has purpose, but that the observer's personal and professional mindset influences its perception and attribution (Burgner, Jirovec, Murrell, & Barton, 1992; English & Morse, 1988; Podrasky & Sexton, 1988). The process of reframing challenges attitudes, values, and responses, resulting in a modified interpretation of a given situation and, thus, a change in behavioral response (Johnson & Werstlein, 1990).

Staff in nonpsychiatric settings often have had minimal preparation to assess, understand, or respond to "difficult" patient behaviors; thus, they attempt to control them from within a medical model (psychoactive drugs and physical restraints) rather than using a more holistic, psychosocial response. Attempting to control the behavior in these ways actually increases the likelihood of iatrogenic problems an exacerbates the "difficult behavior." Such behavior is often a symptom of an underlying illness or an expression of unmet need; thus, exploring reasons for the behavior is imperative. Attention and effective response to these behaviors by the interdisciplinary team actually makes caring more challenging, creative, interesting, and rewarding to caregivers, and contributes to improved health outcomes and quality of life for older adults. A prerequisite is knowing the patient.

Collecting Clues

Knowing the patient permits individualization of care (Jenny & Logan, 1992). Thus, the nurse must learn as quickly as possible the everyday habits, practices and preferences, usual demeanor, and self-presentation of the patient. This will require talking with the patient, family, staff, and other health team members, and developing a liaison with nursing home and home health nurses; reviewing health records; and assessing physical, mental, and functional status, and the environment. An important objective is to identify and respond appropriately to any treatable cause of the behavior, such as infection, dehydration, drug toxicity, sensory deficit, hunger, full bladder, pain. Especially for longer-staying patients, a Behavioral Monitoring Log (Strumpf, Patterson, Evans, & Wagner, 1992) can be used to describe the context or circumstances of the behavior. The Log can help identify who is most affected by the behavior and the When, What, Where, Who, Why, and How of the behavior. Over a number of days, a pattern may be identified. Through examination of the pattern together with the patient's own perception and emotional response, the meaning of the behavior may be derived. A psychiatric-liaison clinical nurse specialist may be an important consultant in this process.

Designing Individualized Responses

Depending on what is learned from the assessment, there may be a range of alternative interventions for the types of "difficult" behaviors. Interventions may be categorized according to physiologic, activity, psychosocial, and environmental strategies (Evans, Strumpf, & Williams, 1992), but the approach should always be individualized. At this stage of our knowledge development, there is no one standard response for each type of need. Research-based alternatives are sparse, although studies on wandering (Algase, 1992), physical aggression (Ryden & Feldt, 1992), and excess disability (Salisbury, 1991) are daily contributing information. Other responses derive from expert clinical practice and common sense. All represent less restrictive measures than immobilization from physical restraints. Frequent orientation, reassurance, obtaining personal items from home, and assignment of consistent caregivers may be effective in helping the confused elder feel safe and secure and, thus, may prevent "difficult" behavior from arising. The remainder of this chapter will focus on fall risk and treatment interference, which are among the most challenging needs in the acute-care setting. (More detailed information regarding responses to these and other needs may be found in Strumpf, Patterson, et al. (1992).)

Fall Risk.   Concerns about fall risk are of three main types: (1) falling while getting out of bed, (2) sliding out of chair, and (3) falling while ambulating. Falls are frequent, nonrandom occurrences among older adults, and their rates are similar among those in and outside of institutions. Most falls do not result in serious injury, suggesting that efforts should be aimed at preventing serious injury from falls, not in preventing all falls. Age-related changes (gait and postural/balance changes), age-associated health problems (peripheral vascular disease, peripheral neuropathy, poor vision), environmental factors (shiny or slippery floors, loose carpet, poor lighting) or other factors (drug side effects) are common causes of falls in the hospital setting. Characteristics of the frequent faller may include advanced age, altered emotional state, relocation, debilitation, visual impairment, altered gait/balance, altered mental status, incontinence, history of falling, confinement to chair, postural hypotension, and medications (Strumpf, Patterson, et al., 1992).

When creative, nonrestrictive interventions are used with frequent fallers, they should be based on an individualized assessment. High-risk identification systems, environmental adapta'tions, and reconditioning programs are important strategies. Depending on the patient's need, safe egress from the bed can be facilitated by such things as a low bed (14 to 18 inches from the floor) or temporary use of a mattress on the floor; nonuse of bedrails or use of half or three-quarter rails; accessible call light; bed/chair alarms; bedside toilet, or assistance in adhering to the patient's usual elimination schedule; nonskid flooring or strips; night lighting; and proper footwear. New design units may consider installing a window to the hallway for selected rooms to permit ease in supervising the status of bed- or chair-bound patients. To prevent a patient with poor muscle tone or strength from sliding from a chair, remedies include a chair that fits the patient, support pillows, nonslip materials such as Dycem (Maddock, Inc., Pequannock, NJ), wedge-shaped or bean bag cushions, use of a wheelchair for transport but not seating, frequent change of position, timely toilet routines, or placing the patient near the nursing station. Daily weight-bearing, a mobility program using proper assistive devices, and orientation to a clearly identified and safe walking path should be employed as soon as possible after admission, to prevent deconditioning.

Interference with Medical Treatment. A person who interferes with medical treatment, such as by pulling out intravenous lines, feeding or tracheostomy tubes, or urinary catheters, presents both clinical challenges and ethical dilemmas. Clinically, the question arises: How can the care deemed necessary to sustain life be provided while the patient is cognitively unable to cooperate? Ethical concerns about burdens and benefits of invasive treatment must consider the patient's advance directives and what is in the best interest of the patient. Prevention of the need for such treatment at the outset may be achieved through attention to physical/psychological status; prompt treatment of underlying medical conditions; and respect for advance directives and treatment choices. Guidelines for care of the person who requires invasive treatments include selecting the least intrusive treatment possible and eliminating the treatment as soon as possible—for example, resuming oral feeding and hydration; repeatedly explaining the treatment to be used, and providing time for guided exploration of the device and site; making the patient comfortable in order to facilitate tolerance of the treatment (e.g., padding of the site) and, if restraint is the only short-term solution, using the least restrictive device. Examples of ways to enable the elder to tolerate short-term use of invasive treatment devices include explanation; camouflage of site; distractors; and use of a family member or paid companion for supervision and orientation. Air splints (Rader & Donius, 1991) or opposition splints are examples of less restrictive devices when some form of restraint is deemed necessary to permit short-term treatment.

In general, the routine use of physical restraints to manage "difficult behavior" represents a poor quality of care. Older adults function and heal best in environments where they feel safe and secure—environments that are homelike, individualized, and normalized. Such environments support reasonable risk taking, respect personal dignity, and enhance quality of life.

REFERENCES

Algase, D. L. (1992). A century of progress: Today's strategies for responding to wandering behavior. *Journal of Gerontological Nursing, 18*(11), 28–34.

Blakeslee, J., Goldman, B., Papougenis, D., & Torell, C. (1991). Making the transition to restraint-free care. *Journal of Gerontological Nursing, 17*(2), 4–8.

Burgner, S. C., Jirovec, M., Murrell, L., & Barton, D. (1992). Caregiver and environmental variables related to difficult behaviors in institutionalized demented elderly persons. *Journal of Gerontology, 47*(4), 242–249.

English, J., & Morse, J. M. (1988). The "difficult" elderly patient: Adjustment or maladjustment? *International Journal of Nursing Studies, 25*(1), 23–39.

English, R. A. (1989). Implementing a non-restraint philosophy. *The Canadian Nurse, 85*(3), 52–55.

Evans, L. K., & Strumpf, N. E. (1989). Tying down the elderly: A review of the literature on physical restraint. *Journal of American Geriatrics Society, 37,* 65–74.

Evans, L. K., & Strumpf, N. E. (1990). Myths about elder restraint. *Image: The Journal of Nursing Scholarship, 22*(2), 124–128.

Evans, L. K., & Strumpf, N. E. (1992). Reducing restraints: One nursing home's story. In S. G. Funk, E. Tornquist, M. Champagne, & R. Wiese (Eds.), *Key aspects of elder care* (pp. 118–128). New York: Springer.

Evans, L. K., Strumpf, N. E., & Williams, C. C. (1992). Limiting use of physical restraints: A prerequisite for independent functioning. In E. Calkins, A. Ford, & P. Katz (Eds.), *Practice of geriatrics* (2nd ed.; pp. 204–210). Philadelphia: Saunders.

Jenny, J., & Logan, J. (1992). Knowing the patient: One aspect of clinical knowledge. *Image: The Journal of Nursing Scholarship, 24*(4), 254–258.

Johnson, G. B., & Werstlein, P. O. (1990). Reframing: A strategy to improve care of manipulative patients. *Issues in Mental Health Nursing, 11,* 237–241.

Joint Commission on Accreditation of Healthcare Organizations (1991). Restraint and seclusion scoring guidelines. *Joint Commission Perspectives,* January/February, Insert, D1–5.

Lofgren, R. P., McPherson, D. S., Granieri, R., Myllenbeck, S., & Sprafka, J. M. (1989). Mechanical restraints on the medical wards: Are protective devices safe? *American Journal of Public Health, 79,* 735–738.

Miles, S. H., & Irvine, P. (1992). Deaths caused by physical restraints. *Gerontologist, 32*(6), 762–766.

Mitchell-Pedersen, L., Fingerote, E., Powell, C., & Edmund, L. (1989). Avoiding restraints: Why it can mean good practice. *Nursing, 19*(9), 66–72.

Nightingale, F. (1859). *Notes on nursing.* Philadelphia: Lippincott.

Podrasky, D. L., & Sexton, D. L. (1988). Nurses' reactions to difficult patients. *Image: The Journal of Nursing Scholarship, 20*(1), 16–21.

Rader, J., & Donius, M. (1991). Leveling off restraints. *Geriatric Nursing, 31*(2), 71–73.

Ryden, M. B., & Feldt, K. S. (1992). Goal-directed care: Caring for aggressive nursing home residents with dementia. *Journal of Gerontologic Nursing, 18*(11), 35–42.

Salisbury, S. A. (1991). Preventing excess disability. In W. C. Chenitz, J. T. Stone, & S. A. Salisbury (Eds.), *Clinical gerontological nursing* (pp. 391–401). Philadelphia: Saunders.

Stone, J. T. (1991). Preventing physical iatrogenic problems. In W. C. Chenitz, J. T. Stone, & S. A. Salisbury (Eds.), *Clinical gerontological nursing* (pp. 359–375). Philadelphia: Saunders.

Strumpf, N. E., & Evans, L. K. (1992). Editorial: Alternatives to physical restraints. *Journal of Gerontological Nursing, 18*(11), 4.

Strumpf, N. E., Evans, L. K., Wagner, J., & Patterson, J. (1992). Reducing physical restraints: Developing an educational program. *Journal of Gerontological Nursing, 18*(11), 21–27.

Strumpf, N. E., Patterson, J., Evans, L. K., & Wagner, J. (1992). *Reducing restraints: Individualized approaches to behavior.* Huntingdon Valley, PA: The Whitman Group.

Strumpf, N. E., & Tomes, N. (1993). Restraining the troublesome patient: A historical perspective on a contemporary debate. *Nursing History Review, 1,* 3–24.

Tappen, R. M., & Beckerman, A. (1992). The hospitalized frail older adult. *Geriatric Nursing, 13*(3), 149–152.

Tinetti, M. E., Liu, W. L., & Ginter, S. F. (1992). Mechanical restraint use and fall-related injuries among residents of skilled nursing facilities. *Annals of Internal Medicine, 116,* 369–374.

Weeks, C. S. (1885). *A textbook of nursing.* New York: Appleton.

Weick, M. D. (1992). Physical restraints: An FDA update. *American Journal of Nursing, 92*(11), 80.

6

Ways of Knowing and Caring for Older Adults

Sister Rosemary Donley

Anyone who reviews the statistics about aging recognizes that America, like countries in Western Europe, is aging. We are no longer surprised to read that the fastest growing segment of our society is over 85. The most dramatic changes in human development occur early in life, but only mature persons can reflect on their own aging process, which is described, variously, as a slowing, a diminishment, a maturation, the golden years, generativity, or loss. Because aging affects the physical, social, spiritual, and intellectual patterns of individuals, it changes human relationships. Many older people fear symptoms that alter their mobility, continence, and cognition because the onset of this triad of symptoms leads to significant disability and eventually to death (Perry & Butler, 1990).

Social factors also contribute to the challenge of growing old. Women, the largest group of elderly persons in America, have outlived their spouses and many of their friends and relatives. New family constellations; the geographic disbursement of families; the number of women, who have been historically the caretakers, now in the workplace; and longevity itself—all contribute to older women living alone or in caretaker relationships with aging siblings (Bunting, 1992). Although fewer elderly than in earlier generations are below the poverty line, aged persons live with fewer resources because incomes are reduced at the time of retirement. Eventually, people on stable incomes are affected by fluctuations in the economy, changes in their neighborhoods, and the uneven buying power of their dollars. Many persons in nursing homes are poor. Minorities face greater social losses as they enter their senior years because of previous economic and social disadvantage. Perhaps the most awesome experience of aging, however, is the loss of importance to others. Older people stand at a liminal point, a threshold of change (Turner, 1974). If the older person's identity has been rooted solely in work, in family, or in social position, or has been invested exclusively in a particular life-style, the ambiguity of the transition into aging can be frightening. To the degree that public policy and private action affirm youth, marginalize the dependent, or alienate the aged, the passage into old age becomes more frightening. Those who understand and care for the older person can link outcomes of care to an older person's experience of liminality and to private actions and public policies that restrict social engagement and independence (Donley, 1993a).

In drawing practical suggestions about ways of caring, I am guided by the principle that caring follows knowing. Informed caregivers know demographic and social data about the particular group or population of older persons under their care. They possess information about their actual and anticipated health status. Knowledgeable caregivers also seek to glimpse the worldview of aged persons as they try to understand how aging individuals perceive their conditions and think about the future. The OBRA*-mandated assessments of residents ("Conditions of Participation . . . ," 1989) were designed to help staff in nursing homes know their clients and plan more individualized care for them. Unfortunately, the attitudinal transformation that underlies movement from ritualistic practice to personalized care cannot be legislated (Walker, 1967). Education of caregivers holds the key to nursing's quest to enhance ways of caring by expanding ways of knowing.

Health care reform addresses many of the issues that gave rise to this conference: cost, access, and quality. However, on examination, the Clinton campaign agenda of managed competition proposed less reform and more revision to the current pattern of financing and regulating health care services. It is too soon to determine which mix of factors will influence presidential and congressional action about the future health care

---

* Omnibus Budget Reconciliation Act (OBRA), Subtitle C, Nursing Home Reform, P. L. 100-203 (1987; effective 1990). Text available from U.S. Government Printing Office, Washington, DC.

system: political concerns, presidential or congressional campaign promises, the aspirations of representatives and senators, the influence of lobbies and special interest groups, constituent complaints, or the issues themselves. If we can set the political agenda aside, the issues are significant. They include the cost of health care, which consumes about 13% of the gross national product; the effect of rising health care costs on the American economy and American competitiveness in the world marketplace; the number of people without health insurance; the disproportionate share of federal and private dollars spent on acute care; the human and financial cost of misuse/overuse/abuse by providers and patients; the costs of regulation; and the quality of services (Blendon et al., 1992). The Clinton agenda will also discuss health care outcomes from an international perspective. Indicators show significant differences in:

- Infant mortality (in 1990, the number of deaths of children under 1 year of age per 1,000 births was 10.4 in the United States, compared with 7.3 in Canada and Britain, 5.9 in Sweden, and 4.5 in Japan;

- Levels of immunization (in the United States, only 70% of 1-year-old children are fully immunized against childhood diseases—diphtheria, measles, and polio; in other First World countries—Sweden, Canada, Japan, and Britain—immunization levels range from 78 to 97%;

- Life expectancy (the average life for Americans is 75.6 years, compared with 79.3 for the Japanese, 79.2 for Canadians, 77.7 for Swedes, and 76.3 for residents of Britain). (Relman, 1992)

Any responsive agenda will need to address almost immediately the serious gaps in health care services for American mothers and children.

Because the major focus of the Clinton health care plan is directed toward lowering costs, improving access, and enhancing the management of the acute-care service delivery systems ("Managed Competition: . . . ," 1993), it can easily be dominated by arguments about the cost of high-technology practices and the funding of Medicare and Medicaid. However, the delivery system, especially the long-term-care delivery system, is also in crisis (Schlesinger & Mechanic, 1993). Over the years, nursing homes and home care programs have benefited from federal funding. Yet, as Collopy, Boyle, and Jennings (1991) have noted, federal dollars from Medicare and Medicaid have carried acute-care priorities, messages, and restrictions. Ironically, the very system established to help the elderly with acute illness has become the stumbling block to the development of an informed, comprehensive system of quality care delivery for the aged and chronically ill.

Caring follows knowing. Persons who wish to influence health care reform must demonstrate new methods of delivering care, improving outcomes, and lowering costs. New networks and coalitions must be established with consumers and the business community. This is not a call to reinvent the wheel. There are good models of cost-effective care delivery; they need to be replicated, promoted, and publicized (Barger, 1991, Bower, 1992, Korman, 1991). Public policy makers need to be informed of these innovative care systems so that the new agenda for health care supports preventive and primary care services in addition to building on the experience of Medicare and Medicaid.

Discussions about the nature of caring relationships address the subject of curing on the way to discourses about care. Sometimes, curing is set up in an adversarial position to caring. The cure-versus-care formulation describes the tension between the scientific rigor of high-technology medicine and the more holistic efforts to touch the inner spirit and lifestyle of the person. Cure seeks the eradication of disease. Its ethic is the therapeutic imperative. For the curer, no cost or burden is too great if it advances medical science's ability to cure. Caring is more intuitive. Guided by creative imagination and spiritual insight, caring uses touch, communication, compassion, insight, and empathy to heal the diseased person. Caring has not been easy to define in operational or budget-oriented terms. It seems to be dependent on the actions of virtuous, knowledgeable persons and the relational contexts in which the caring actions take place. The positive outcomes of caring actions may not diminish disease processes. However, these outcomes are often the subjective experience of symptom relief or the liberation of the person from suffering. Recently, writers have begun to discuss cure and care from moral perspectives, speaking about an ethic of cure and an ethic of care (Gadow, 1988). In this context, caring is described as a covenant and "the commitment to alleviating another's vulnerability" (pp. 6–7).

In practice, however, cure cannot be separated from care. The Picker Commonwealth Program for Patient-Centered Care (*Picker/Commonwealth Report*, 1992) demonstrates this point in its longitudinal study of acutely ill, hospitalized persons. The report states unequivocally that emotional support is integral to the patient's sense of well-being and to good patient care outcomes. It also notes that caring is more complex than hand-holding and reassurance.

Cure can be placed in an adversarial relationship to care in discussions about funding of research, investment in alternate delivery systems, and support for training and payment of health providers who are not physicians. In the United States, powerful medical, drug, hospital, and medical supply lobbies work against any legislation or policy that threatens their influence and diminishes the income they extract from the acute health care system. In times of cost containment, priorities of cure compete with and hold back the advancement of the care agenda. These allocation debates are now on center stage as concerns about health care costs have called into question the cost, benefit, and burden of high-technology medicine (Eddy, 1991). Callahan (1988) has focused the debate more sharply by asking how much treatment should be directed toward the elderly.

Medical wisdom has assumed that patients will opt for the ethic of cure and choose those research and clinical initiatives that promise cure or longevity. These assumptions have guided medical practice and decision making. However, Wennberg's (1990) research suggests that patients may be more conservative than their physicians and prefer "watchful waiting" to intervention. A new federal initiative, the Self Determination Act of 1991, the so-called "right to know legislation," requires that health care providers consult with patients, presenting and explaining the benefits and burdens of proposed medical interventions before they are initiated, changed, or continued.

"Care" is rarely presented as an equal or real option to cure. Care is portrayed as "second best"—a response to painful human situations that can be evoked if all else fails or if treatment is found to be wanting. Several years ago, in the presentation of the Shattuck lecture in *The New England Journal of Medicine,* Wheeler (1990) noted that the medical and public press ignored or underreported research about care. He noted studies in which participation in a support group, when coupled with standard therapy for breast cancer, was shown to extend significantly the lives of women. He also reported that men with myocardial infarctions had better survival rates when they enjoyed supportive personal relationships.

Care initiatives have not been developed or tested as well as their high-technology counterparts; research about caring activities is underfunded and underreported; persons who provide care or who study and teach caring processes and outcomes are assigned peripheral roles in the health professional hierarchy; and caring acts are undervalued (Gordon, 1991). Given the competitiveness and self-interest of many in the health care field, caring has not had a fair market test. Because knowing precedes caring, more information and knowledge about caring needs to emerge from nursing theory and nursing research.

Several months ago, I was asked to prepare a paper about quality in long-term care nursing education. In that paper, I proposed that quality (excellence) in long-term care could be approached by studying caring relationships between persons (Donley, 1993b). This formulation examined the caring action, the result brought about by the caring action, and the effect of the action upon the person who performed it.

Caring actions can be observed, described, demonstrated, changed, and evaluated. The effects or outcomes of these caring actions can also be measured because they are reflected in changes in the well-being and quality of life of the person who received the care. Caring activities engage the caregiver in a human relationship, which influences the self-esteem and sense of personal fulfillment of the caregivers. These changes can be described and measured. Because knowing is a prelude to caring, I propose a research agenda for the care of the aged based on these three aspects of the caring relationship: (1) the act of care itself, (2) the outcome of the act, and (3) the effect of the action on the person who performed it. This construct will serve not only to increase knowledge about aged persons, but also to provide a framework for teaching and learning about care of older persons.

REFERENCES

Barger, S. (1992). The nursing center: A model for rural nursing practice. *Nursing and Health Care, 12*(6), 290–294.

Blendon, R. J., Altman, D. E., Benson, J. M., Taylor, H., James, M., & Smith, M. (1992). The implication of the 1992 presidential election for health care reform. *Journal of the American Medical Association, 268*(23), 3371–3375.

Bower, K. A. (1992). *Case management by nurses.* Washington, DC: American Nurses Association.

Bunting, S. M. (1992). Eve's legacy: An analysis of family caregiving from a feminist perspective. In J. Thompson, D. Allen, & L. Rodriques-Fisher (Eds.), *Critique, resistance, and action* (pp. 53–68). New York: National League for Nursing.

Callahan, D. (1988). Setting limits: Medical goals in an aging society. In J. Watson & M. A. Ray (Eds.), *The ethics of care and the ethics of cure: Synthesis in chronicity* (pp. 15–19). New York: National League for Nursing.

Collopy, B., Boyle, P., & Jennings, B. (1991, March–April). New directions in nursing home ethics. *Hasting Center Report* (Special Supplement), 1–15.

Conditions of participation and requirements for long-term care facilities. (1989, February 2). *Federal Register, 54*(21), 5353–5373.

Donley, R. (1993a). Not the weak of heart: The politics of long-term care. In M. Burke & S. Sherman (Eds.), *Gerontological nursing: Issues and opportunities for the twenty-first century* (pp. 1–12). New York: National League for Nursing.

Donley, R. (1993b). The relationship of quality in long-term care nursing education. In E. L. Mitty (Ed.), *Quality imperatives in long-term care: The illusive agenda* (pp. 7–12). New York: National League for Nursing.

Eddy, D. M. (1991, February 13). What care is "essential"? What services are basic? *Journal of the American Medical Association,* X(X), 782–788.

Gadow, S. (1993). Covenant without cure: Letting go and holding on in chronic illness. In J. Watson & M. A. Ray (Eds.), *Ethics of care* (pp. 5–14). New York: National League for Nursing.

Gordon, S. (1991, January). A national care agenda. *The Atlantic Monthly,* 64–68.

Korman, R. (1991). Bedside terminals can improve nursing efficiency. *Health Care Financial Management, 45*(4), 48 ff.

Managed competition: Health reform American style (Supplement). (1993). *Health Affairs, 12,* 5–299.

Perry, D., & Butler, R. (1990). Aim not just for longer life but expanded "health span." In P. Homer & M. Holstein (Eds.), *A good old age?* (pp. 91–94). New York: Simon & Schuster.

Picker/Commonwealth Report (pp. 1–8). (1992, Winter). Boston: Beth Israel Hospital.

Relman, A. S. (August, 1992). Reforming our health care system: A physician's perspective. *The Key Reporter, 58*(1), 1–6. Washington, DC: Phi Beta Kappa.

Schlesinger, M., & Mechanic, D. (1993). Challenges for managed competition from chronic illness. *Health Affairs* (Supplement), *12,* 123–137.

Turner, V. (1974). *Dramas, fields and metaphors.* Ithaca: Cornell University Press.

Walker, V. (1967). *Nursing and ritualistic practice.* New York: MacMillan.

Wennberg, J. E. (1990). Outcomes research, cost containment and the fear of health care rationing. *New England Journal of Medicine, 323,* 1202–1204.

Wheeler, H. B. (1990, May 24). Shattuck lecture: Healing and heroism. *New England Journal of Medicine, 332,* 1540–1548.

7

Parallel Worlds of Nursing Practice

Elaine Tagliareni, Andrea Mengel, and Susan Sherman

I work nights on a medical unit. We have a long-term patient; his name is Henry. He is in his late 80s. He is in and out a lot—four times in the year I've worked there. He has a history of congestive heart failure, chronic obstructive pulmonary disease, and diabetes. Henry has never been especially compliant with his treatment. We know him well. The last time he came in he was really bad. For three nights he was in and out of congestive heart failure; it was touch and go. By the fourth day, he began coming out of it—walking a bit but always short of breath. I began to say to myself, "I think Henry is going to make it." I felt good. After Henry had been there about seven days, he was ready for discharge again. I was making rounds about midnight and Henry wasn't in his room. I knew where to go. I found him in the unit kitchen, searching for saltines and ice cream. He looked at me and I looked at him and we smiled. I thought to myself, "You did a good job Brian; Henry's back!"

> Brian Jones,
> Class of 1992
> Community College of Philadelphia

Brian Jones is a recent graduate of the nursing program at Community College of Philadelphia (CCP). Brian told his story about Henry during a focus group session of graduates, held at the college. The focus group participants represented graduates practicing in both acute-care and long-term care environments. All of them had graduated from CCP during the department's involvement in the W.K. Kellogg-sponsored Community College–Nursing Home Partnership project, and all had participated in a nursing curriculum that included a second-level nursing home rotation as well as focused learning activities that addressed the special needs of the older adult.

As faculty members at CCP, we organized focus group sessions with a twofold purpose: (1) to describe the experience of providing nursing care to older adults in both acute-care and long-term care settings; and (2) to identify experiences at CCP that best prepared graduates for effective practice in their present work environments. The focus group discussions were structured to be informal and spontaneous. As all sessions were opened, attendees were asked to describe their nursing practice with older adults. (See 7.1.)

Brian's story, like many others we heard from fifteen graduates over the course of three sessions, is telling. Brian accepted Henry for who he was and how he viewed the world. Brian understood that getting better, for Henry, meant not only resolution of his cardiac failure and fluid overload but also included Henry's return to saltines and ice cream. When Brian told his story, he discussed the staff's reactions to Henry's wanderings. "They were angry," he said. "They said, 'Henry should know better. He'll never get better if he doesn't change his diet. He'll be right back in here again.'" Brian's ability to be subjective and personalized in a world that is so often objective and ritualized, and his conviction that Henry had achieved wellness on his own terms, a belief not generally accepted in today's acute-care driven health care settings, challenged us to reflect on his words and to discover meaning in his story.

Brian, it seemed to us, had developed a paradigm for nursing practice that transcended setting. Brian works in the high-technology, high-stimulus world of acute care, where cure-oriented methodologies predominate and where older individuals, like Henry, are often labeled noncompliant when their belief system conflicts with current, accepted practice. Yet, Brian and his classmates view their practice differently. When we asked Brian to describe a powerful nursing moment, he chose to talk about Henry, and about how he had helped Henry back to wellness, on Henry's terms. The significance of Brian's story lies in his willingness to value Henry's history and accept Henry's sense of "being in the world."

Perhaps, we thought, this perspective had its origins in the long-term care clinical experience where the practice patterns of the nursing home environment are studied and known: to assist individuals to function

Figure 7.1
Focus Group Discussion Questions

Describe your practice.

What story from your clinical practice, especially with older adults, had special meaning for you?

Tell us about a day when you left the unit and said, "Today was a good day." Tell us about a moment during the day when you said to yourself, "I did a good job."

What issues in your daily practice have the most impact on you?

What makes an experience rewarding for you? Is your job rewarding? Tell us about a rewarding experience.

---

optimally in a safe and familiar environment; to foster rehabilitation potential in each person, despite multiple chronic illnesses and concomitant cognitive and functional disabilities; and to value older adults as persons with dignity, whose belief systems and past experiences are significant determinants of present reality. How, we asked, are the practice patterns from the nursing home reflected in Brian's story? What are the differences between the nurse's work in acute-care and long-term care settings? What is the essential nature of the nurse's work in both settings?

Taking cues from phenomenological research methodology, we transcribed on index cards statements made by group participants, and then, independently, arranged the cards according to themes that characterized the group's experience in acute care and long-term care. By attending to the special meanings in the experiences of the graduates, we reflected on their stories, confirmed them, and used them as the basis for the theory of the parallel worlds of nursing. The literature on ways of knowing and the ideas presented by Holly Skodol Wilson at this conference gave us permission and validation to draw on the clinical knowledge of nurses in specific contexts and to use that knowledge to inform the practice of teaching and the ways of caring. This knowledge, always personal and subjective, is an essential foundation for nursing and is the specialized knowledge gained through experiences in practice situations.

What emerged from our deliberations of the focus group dialogue is a working model to understand the nature of nurses' work in long-term care and acute-care settings (Figure 7.2), called "Parallel Worlds of Nursing Practice." We theorized that the parallel worlds in acute care and long-term care reflect different institutional values and ethics, and that the nature of the nurses' work in each setting varies. We also concluded, from stories like Brian's, that powerful nursing moments occurred when graduates merged the knowledge and values from both worlds into a personal practice paradigm.

SETTING

Early in our experience with the Community College–Nursing Home Partnership, we understood that the setting of the nursing home, where the focus of care is on activities of daily living, rehabilitation, recreational and diversional activities, and promotion of quality of living, provides opportunities for students to plan nursing care that is primarily directed toward promotion and maintenance of optimal functional ability, rehabilitation potential, and improved well-being, regardless of the individual's cure potential. We realized that this perspective contrasted sharply with the focus of care in the acute setting. This realization led us to design, in the nursing home, learning objectives that highlighted these differences. Recognizing the importance of assisting students to create therapeutic environments in a nonacute, nontechnologically oriented setting, we

Figure 7.2
A Model to Understand the Nature of Nurses' Work in Acute Care and Long-Term Care Settings

PARALLEL WORLDS OF NURSING PRACTICE

Transition Setting Ex. Acute Care	Homelike Setting Ex. The Nursing Home
Ritualistic practice, specialized care planning focusing on a crisis event. Interventions are standardized and sporadic.	Personalized practice, comprehensive care planning within the context of current and past life events. Interventions are individualized and continuous.
Goals relate to resolution of acute, identified problems using technology and efficiency.	Goals relate to assisting individuals to function optimally in a safe and familiar environment.
Rewards derive from making connections with patients in the context of helping them to get better or die well.	Rewards derive from knowing individuals over time, maximizing potential, and improving the quality of the living environment.

**A successful core of nursing practice occurs
when the nurse exercises the choice and the
self-confidence to merge the knowledge
and the values learned in both settings into a
personal practice paradigm.**

selected concepts about nursing that could not be taught as well in the hospital setting. We set out to teach students to orient their thinking and care planning toward the promotion of health and well-being in an environment that is safe and familiar, an environment where cure-oriented interventions and disease treatment modalities may, in fact, shortchange the Henrys of this world, who seek to be cared for in an environment that supports living and dignified decline (Waters, 1991, p. 23). During the years of project activities, we began to call this environment "homelike."

Conversely, we continually referred to the acute-care setting as a world "seized by technology" (Boyd, 1988), a world characterized by standardized treatment protocols, high acuity, and shortened length of stay. When a partnership faculty member described acute care as a "transitional setting, no longer a landing place for cure" (Tagliareni, 1992, p. 32), we were captured by the nursing implications inherent in this perspective. We realized that the transitional environment of acute care was fundamentally different from the acute-care environment in which we had grown and developed as practitioners and faculty members. We had known a world where patients came in to be prepared for surgery and stayed to convalesce. We had experienced a world where we knew patients for 2 to 3 weeks and were able to evaluate progress in light of personal events. The new world of acute care is different and requires new approaches to care planning in a short-stay, high-stimulus environment. As we listened to participants in the focus groups, and analyzed their statements, we became aware of clear differences between the "homelike" setting of the nursing home and the "transitional" setting of acute care. The experiences described by the focus group participants revealed a striking contrast between the two settings in the areas of practice patterns, goal setting, and rewarding encounters.

PRACTICE PATTERNS

Through the focus group discussions, a core of nursing practice emerged. It included: providing direct patient care, advocating for basic human needs, and valuing interpersonal moments between the nurse and the client and family.

> If I had to do something that was just technical and I couldn't talk and touch and make them [patients] laugh, I would be out of nursing.
>
> You start little by little. You become the most essential person to that family and that is what I like. You keep it all together for them.
>
> Patients have a lot of fears. You need time to talk with them. Talking with them makes the difference.
>
> In the CCU, an older woman was screaming. She had a very irritating voice. Everyone dismissed her as old and agitated—hopeless. It was frustrating. But I stayed with her and said, "You are with me; you are safe" and she stopped.

Earlier in this conference, when discussing caring encounters in nursing, Sister Rosemary Donley charged us to move from ritualistic practice to personalized care. We are intrigued by her words because, after analysis of the focus group data, we realized that ritualistic versus personalized accurately contrasts caregiving in acute care and in the nursing home.

Standardization of care planning and specialized interventions directed toward specific events emerged as a theme describing nursing practice in acute-care settings.

I don't like being a task master, just doing protocols. I'd like to have more time talking and finding out needs.

There are so many things that are policy, like calling for a blood sugar. I can make that judgment, about giving O.J., and I have to call the doctor. I thought more things would be nursing judgment. Lots of routine orders.

We have standardized care plans and you just highlight the parts that fit your patient.

Conversely, individualization and creativity were frequently mentioned as outcomes in long-term care. Each event, each caring situation, is unique, and interventions require a knowledge of the resident that includes the individual's history of significant life events, previous responses to caregivers and to the living environment, and medical and nursing management. "Routine" exists only in relation to institutional protocols. The nurse's response to residents and to changing events is subjective and often involves intuition.

In the nursing home you can talk with the residents. If one of them is having a problem, you can try to work it out. It is never the same. That's what you expect. People are agitated and confused and you just go ahead and deal with it.

People constantly say that long-term care nursing is not creative. I'd like them to come up with ideas about how to keep a resident from wandering away!

Sometimes you have a gut feeling about something. You are waiting for the resident to do something that is more definite. He just doesn't look right. It's a gut feeling.

Another theme in focus group discussions was the ambiguous nature of decision making in both the acute-care and long-term care environments. Graduates expected a more structured, objective approach to nursing care delivery, and often expressed frustration.

In critical care, decisions about ethics are not clear—the gray area is wider all the time. Things are supposed to be clear but they aren't. It's easy to make ethical decisions in class but it's hard in reality.

I think that the job in acute care is clearer and the job in long-term care is fuzzy . . . the boundaries are not clear. The jobs are so many and varied.

To put someone on a feeding tube when they don't want it is not quality of life and yet it happens all the time. If someone is ready to accept death and they have lived a full life, then let them make the decision to die. I accept that, but sometimes we can't do what patients want.

During the keynote address, Holly Skodol Wilson spoke about shaping chaos as a way of knowing. She challenged us to rethink our premise that the world is linear and facts and principles exist noncontextually. Perhaps the world is orderly and chaotic simultaneously. We know the current world of health care is characterized by ambiguity, complexity, and uncertainty. Yet, students often graduate from nursing programs with the belief that nursing outcomes are well-defined and clearly prescribed. As nurse educators, we need to ask ourselves whether our current teaching methodologies, often passive and authoritarian, and our operationalization of the nursing process in the form of linear, problem-focused care plans, limit the students' view of the world of nursing and health care. Understanding the lived experiences of illness and frailty escapes the formalization of the traditional nursing care plan approach (Tanner, 1988). We have come to realize that nursing practice in the nursing home may in fact provide students with a different lens to view health care. The view through this new lens allows students to challenge assumptions and discover a context for their new knowledge.

Providing nursing care today, in any setting, requires a willingness to embrace ambiguity, to develop care plans that address individualized agendas, and to do both in a world engulfed in cure-oriented solutions. As educators, we must seek out less structured environments where outcomes are not readily apparent and ritualized, and we must help students accept ambiguity and uncertainty as natural parts of clinical practice. We believe that we must provide students with experiences in homelike settings, where they can plan care that is personal and individualized and that takes into account cultural, social, and personal contexts.

GOAL SETTING

The theme of advocacy for older adults surfaced in each focus group discussion. For graduates, advocacy became a mission: to understand an older person's behavior and then to explain it in a way that is acceptable and sanctioned by nursing peers, an interpretation that makes sense of the older adults' special way of being in the world. We were surprised by the intensity of indignation in their voices as they talked about the "label" of confusion and the stigma of old age in a world that often treats older adults as objects or stereotypes.

What is the date anyway? To so many of my patients, that is an unfair question. If they know the season after they have been on the unit for weeks, then I check them as correct for orientation to time. . . . When they are sick, all they care about is family. They don't care about the date. I understand that.

You go into a patient's room and ask him a couple of questions and the patient doesn't say the logical thing. But you tell him to move, sit up and he does and the patient will say your name and know you are the nurse and that he is in the hospital; that doesn't equal confusion to me. I always argue with nurses about calling a patient "confused."

I will not call a patient "confused" just because he doesn't say what I wanted him to say right away. With older adults, you need to think about what is most important to them. Why do they need to know the date right now?

When I send residents to the hospital, from the nursing home, I try to write a thorough note about what they can do and how well they understand directions—things like that. And, it makes me so angry that they always come back labeled "confused."

We are constantly working with attitudes, negative attitudes. In the ER, nurses call nursing home residents "gomers." What right do people have to call them that?

I did have a patient who was really confused. Later that morning, I asked the patient to do things for me and he did them—really well. So I wrote a note that his confusion was transient.

While advocacy transcended both settings, distinctions related to goal setting in acute care and long-term care were evident. When describing the nature of the work in acute care, participants spoke about dealing with multiple tasks simultaneously:

You have four to five patients who all have two to three IVs and tons of meds. Sometimes your whole day can be frustrated by waiting for meds

*from the pharmacy or not finding isolation gowns. You go home and you
wonder if you forgot a pill or a treatment.*

Participants also focused on the problem-specific nature of task completion, and expressed concern about the resulting inability "to be a caring nurse."

*At times, I just run around doing one thing after another. You hope that
no one needs anything extra or that you don't get an admission or have
a patient go bad.*

*Sometimes, I feel frustrated that I don't have time to do what I was
taught to do. The hectic pace is trying. I feel like a robot, doing IVs,
meds . . . all those tasks can take most of the day, it can be very disjointed; you just focus on segments of the person.*

*In acute care, you often really don't have time to do little things. Sometimes, I'm not sure which is more important to the dying patient—
another antibiotic or a hair wash.*

It seems that the nature of the transitional setting of acute care is such that the nurse's involvement is primarily in a crisis mode, and an ability to handle technology is essential. In long-term care, the nature of the home-like setting requires a shift in thinking, away from cure-directed outcomes to a focus on the living environment, to promotion of optimal functioning for the resident and creation of a safe milieu that fosters familiarity and genuine concern.

*We deal in a holistic way. I am a technician, social worker, comedian,
manager, friend, counselor. That is what I expected in nursing. Whatever it takes to help them live better, to be content.*

*In the nursing home, there is much more accountability. You are responsible for the nursing care of 45 people who depend on you. You have to
think about all of them when making decisions. It's really important;
they have no one else to count on.*

*We had a resident who kept saying she couldn't walk and she refused to
eat, except when her daughter came, which wasn't all that much. I was
really worried about her. It took time, but she walks now. We are all
really proud of her.*

*Helping people to function to their maximum and helping the family cope
with the situation, that's the challenge.*

Throughout the discussions of goal setting in long-term care, graduates also talked about task completion, especially treatments and paperwork.

Their stories characteristically focused on outcomes that related to assisting older adults to be in a place that promoted optimal daily living, where cure-oriented interventions were less visible and less valued.

REWARDING ENCOUNTERS

One of the key questions asked of the focus group participants related to their perception of rewarding moments in nursing. Initially, we asked them to tell us about a day when they returned home and thought, "Today was a good day." We were awed by the graduates' inability to fully answer this question. "A whole day that was good? I don't think that has ever happened to me." When we edited the question to focus on "rewarding moments," participants easily thought of patient stories. The theme embedded in these stories was the establishment of authentic relationships with patients and residents. Benner and Wrubel (1989) have told us that the act of caring for an individual is synonymous with relationship and that the enabling condition of connection and concern is paramount to caring situations. This sense of connection and concern, always in the context of the human encounter, pervaded the graduates' stories.

Differences in relationship building between the two settings relate to the length of the encounter and to the intent of the interaction. In the acute-care setting, graduates felt rewards when one of two outcomes occurred: (1) when the patient's problem was successfully resolved and the patient "gets better," or (2) when the nurse assists the patient to "die in a caring environment with family and friends." It seemed that rewarding moments occurred when participants made connections with patients and families for an hour or a few days in the context of curing the identified problem, "getting better," or helping the patient accept finality, "dying well."

We had a patient with pneumonia and a pacemaker. He was a DNR. Three nights in a row he went into CHF. On the final day, when he went home, we just looked at him and said, "We did it; we got him out of here." It was amazing to see.

Every time you catch a patient going bad and you save them and they get better, you think "Boy, I really do know something. I'm pretty good."

To help with discharge planning when they are really afraid, feeling that you helped them through it and if it works out and they get better and go home, well, that is the greatest reward.

I work evenings on a medical unit. I saw a patient going down the hall one night and he started to cry. He was dying. So I stopped to talk to him. We sat for a long time. He had always been miserable but then he changed. After that, he always looked for me.

I was working nights and a patient started talking about death. I spent an hour with him, talking about his experience. I got him through it.

Once I talked to a lady about her husband who was dying. She was weeping and I was washing him. She came in, crying. I held her hand and talked. They need to have someone see them through it. I felt good about being there.

In the long-term care environment, emphasis was on knowing the resident over time and facilitating well-being, taking into account the residents' previous life events and current rehabilitation potentials.

One day I was walking by a room of a new resident who had been abused when she lived at home. She started rambling and becoming agitated and I was able to get her to nap after I talked to her. I felt good that she was smiling. I don't think she had smiled much before.

Feedback is a reward. If someone says, "You helped my mother. She is learning to accept it here. I don't know what we would have done." Well, you feel terrific.

The best part for me is knowing the residents. You look at them as people, who they are now, who they were.

Additionally, in the nursing home, gratifying work often involved having an impact on the total living environment, rather than limiting rewards to individual patient encounters.

I've made changes. Only three residents are restrained and only seven residents are on psychotropic meds; I really can make a difference.

When residents were sent all the time to the hospital and didn't really need to go and then were mistreated in the ER, I got administration in the nursing home to change the policy about ER transfer.

In both acute and long-term care, it is evident that developing caring relationships is central to finding reward in the work of nurses. The content of that caring encounter may differ by setting and this difference may contribute to job satisfaction and selection of work environments.

Perhaps the curriculum implication in these graduates' stories relates to assisting students to value the work of nurses in both settings. More specifically, we must help students value well-being and improved functional performance as highly as they regard resolution of time-specific crisis events. Both outcomes are an integral part of nursing practice; both outcomes have meaning and relevance in both acute care and long-term care. The key for students and graduates is in determining the outcome that is the most caring at any given moment, regardless of the setting.

This concept became more significant when we reflected on the large number of rewarding stories that described "dying well" experiences in acute care. In fact, most accounts of truly individualizing care in acute care involved the "dying" experience. Somewhere along the way, graduates had learned that technical skills and task completion are primary until the patient is dying; then it is acceptable and valuable to suspend those crisis-oriented interventions, and focus on comfort and well-being. As educators, we need to help students affirm this shift in thinking and encourage them, when nursing a dying patient, to care more about comfort than about decreased cardiac output.

The basis of caring is knowing another individual in a unique way and that is the reward that sustains nurses, regardless of the setting. Brian knew that. But even more, Brian recognized the value of accepting Henry's view of the world in order to maximize his potential and ensure continuity, rather than defining success totally in relation to cure-oriented standards. Brian found special meaning in knowing Henry, and, in the context of that one encounter, accepted an outcome for Henry that promoted connection and well-being and "getting better." For Henry, that connection had to be subjective and personal.

SUMMARY

During the focus group discussions, Brian described morning rounds:

I was there [on the medical–surgical unit], working 11–7 about 3 months when I realized that by 5 o'clock A.M. practically all of the patients were awake. Most of them were elderly. It wasn't long before I realized that I'd better do something about them being awake. So I made a big pot of coffee and I started bringing coffee around during the 5 A.M. rounds. They really liked it.

When we asked Brian to discuss why he considered coffee at 5 A.M. to be a significant intervention, he replied, "Well, if they were at home, they could get their own coffee." Brian understood the transitional nature of the acute-care setting. He recognized that the older adults on his unit were there only for a brief moment in time and that their personal world must be accounted for when planning nursing care, if that care is to be individualized and comprehensive.

The focus group stories have taught us that nurses must not allow the institutional ethos and values of a setting, whether acute care or long-term care, to impose limitations on their vision of nursing practice. "The role of the nurse," said another focus group participant, "is really to help patients get themselves back to where they consider themselves well again. It's their idea, not ours." From our graduates, we have learned that the parallel worlds of acute-care nursing and long-term care nursing have different characteristics and values and that the nature of the nurse's work in each setting varies. We have also learned to value highly the work of nurses in both settings and to acknowledge that the practice patterns and goal setting from both worlds must be internalized by students if they are to be truly, responsive, health care providers both today and tomorrow.

Unfortunately, in the history of nursing, the problem-specific, crisis-oriented, acute-care model has too often defined curricula and driven our practice. Sadly, we have too often equated increased technology with complexity of care planning, rather than recognizing that care plans, which account for history and promote well-being, are often more complicated and not based solely on rituals and standardized protocols. Perhaps it is time to see things differently and discover new models to describe nursing practice by reflecting on the nature of the nurse's work in both acute and long-term care settings. And, perhaps, by providing students with clinical experiences in homelike settings to complement their acute-care exposure in senior-level courses, we can expand their worldview by teaching them to understand and value the work of nurses in both settings and assist them to develop a personal practice paradigm that incorporates the knowledge and values of both settings. As students enter a world of nursing that demands proficiency in technological skills and standardized protocols while advocating individualized care planning and subjective knowing, we must help them successfully merge the knowledge and skills from parallel worlds into a personal practice paradigm. We believe that the experiences of Brian and his cohorts in the nursing home contributed to their understanding of personalized care in transition settings.

Over the past few years, we have asked ourselves, "How does our presence in the nursing home with students, during a senior-level clinical experience, affect their practice?" We now have a clearer vision. We know we are there not because students will learn essential facts about older adults, although that does occur; not because the need for nursing home beds and community-based health care agencies in this country will increase dramatically in the next twenty to thirty years, and the demand for primary care health providers will rise concomitantly, although that will occur (Pew Health Professions Commission, 1991, pp. 70–72); but because we now understand that to be competent, health-promoting caregivers both today and tomorrow, we must perceive the patient, the focus of our concern, in new ways. We must recognize that the individual who enters the transitional world of acute care seeks well-being and maximum functional ability, as well as cure-oriented, specific interventions. Conversely, the resident who chooses to live in a homelike setting, like the nursing home, often requires resolution of an acute specific problem but more importantly, seeks to be known over time and to feel safe in a familiar and personalized world. With the power of our new insight, we ask you to reflect on the outcomes of the focus groups and to merge the knowledge and the values from the parallel worlds to reconceptualize nursing practice and nursing education.

REFERENCES

Benner, P., & Wrubel, J. (1989). *The primacy of caring.* Menlo Park, CA: Addison-Wesley.

Boyd, C. D. (1988). Phenomenology: A foundation for nursing curriculum. In *Curriculum revolution: Mandate for change* (pp. 65–87). New York: National League for Nursing.

Pew Health Professions Commission. (1991). *Healthy America: Practitioners for 2005.* Durham, NC: Pew Commission.

Tanner, C. (1988). Book Special: Curriculum revolution: The practice mandate. *Nursing and Health Care, 9,* 427–430.

Tagliareni, E. (1993). Issues and recommendations for associate degree education in gerontological nursing. In X. X. Heine (Ed.), *Determining the future of gerontological nursing education* (pp. 60–63). New York: National League for Nursing.

Waters, V. (Ed.). (1991). *Teaching gerontology.* New York: National League for Nursing.

8

Knowing and Caring for
Older People at Home

Barbara K. Haight

THE PROBLEM

Applying today's knowledge to caring for older people at home is a huge task, because home health care has grown exponentially in the past few years. In a recent article proclaiming the success of CHAP (Community Health Accreditation Program, Inc.), Mitchell (1992) highlighted the growth of home care as big business. She noted that Medicare spending on home health care increased by 440% during the 1980s and that 1 in 25 Medicare recipients receives home health services. According to the Bureau of Labor Statistics, home care growth tripled that of the overall health care industry.

In any big business, especially one with such growth, there is usually an influx of entrepreneurs interested chiefly in the outcome dollars. CHAP and the National League for Nursing (NLN) are to be commended for recognizing the need to develop standards and certification guidelines while growth was happening, and for taking part in the policy setting of home care. This may be a first for nursing and it will assure nurses' right to provide quality home care.

The population of older people receiving home care is particularly interesting, both because they have special needs and because they are the largest consumers of home health care. They also can pay their bills, because they have Medicare insurance. In this age of the uninsured, their ability to pay makes older people attractive and sought-after patients, particularly among entrepreneurs whose concern is chiefly an economic outcome.

To guard against a "service-for-money mentality" and to maintain quality nursing care, home care nurses must have knowledge of the special needs of older people, their greatest consumers. Older people who receive home health services usually have functional difficulties and some chronic illnesses. However, just being old does not make one a consumer of home health services. For example, one lady of my acquaintance just celebrated her 80th birthday. She spends 3 days a week volunteering in a hospital; she works at the computer and serves as a patient escort, pushing patients in wheelchairs to their destinations. She considers it good exercise. On her days off, she cares for her own six-room house on a half-acre of land. Two years ago, she hired her first helper, someone to mow the lawn. At present, she is not a recipient of home care, but her future may require at-home services.

A report from the National Medical Expenditure study stated that, in 1987, 14 million people over age 65 had some difficulty performing daily activities (U.S. Department of Health and Human Services, 1992a). The study used measures to examine both ADLs (activities of daily living—tasks essential to basic hygiene) and IADLs (instrumental activities of daily living—tasks used in performing household and social activities). For ADLs, the study found that most older people had difficulty bathing and walking. For IADLs, the greatest problem was transportation in the community. Females were more functionally disabled than males and, of course, functional disability increased with age. African Americans, persons who live alone, and persons on Medicaid were subgroups with the highest percentages of at least one difficulty (U.S. Department of Health and Human Services, 1992b). The medical expenditure survey also examined the patterns of use of community and home services for functionally disabled older people. They found that at least 20% of these people required home care, and although they used other services, they did not use them as extensively (U.S. Department of Health and Human Services, 1992c). Figure 8.1 shows problems with both ADLs and IADLs.

PROVIDERS

To understand the whole scope of the problem, one also must look at the providers. Nursing providers of home health care are not as educated as

Figure 8.1
Problems with Both ADLs and IADLs
Noninstitutionalized Elderly with ADL and Walking Difficulties, 1987.

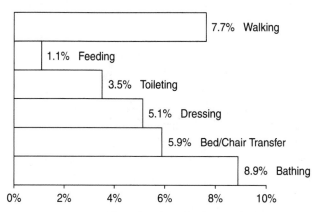

The most common ADL problem for the elderly was bathing, and a considerable number had difficulty walking.

Noninstitutionalized Elderly with IADL Difficulties, 1987.

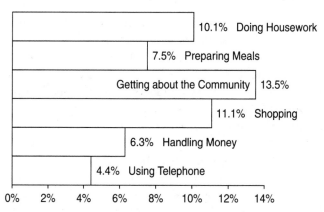

Getting about the community, shopping, and doing housework were the IADL tasks that most frequently caused problems for the elderly.

Adapted from AHCPR Report No. 12.

they should be. Many licensed practical nurses (LPNs) work in home health care with little supervision and low pay. In an article about the dilemma for LPNs who find themselves practicing out in the community with no resources or supervision, one LPN said, "My training was very confusing. Procedures were taught, but not principles. We are left on our own too quickly" (Savorgnani, Haring, & Galloway, 1992). This statement truly illustrates the dilemma of providers in home health care. They not only need further training in skills and procedures, they need background in gerontological nursing.

There are efforts to meet the needs of nurses poorly prepared to care for older people at home. One nursing education program actually provides home care to people who do not qualify for regularly covered services by sending students and instructors to the home to give the needed care (Alster & Keshian, 1990). In Montana, universities make a great effort to provide gerontologic education through outreach efforts and traveling classes (Cudney, 1992). In England, Betts (1987) has presented a very useful scheme using nurse aides to care for elderly people at home. The majority of the recipients of care (70%) in Betts's study felt the nurse aides had enabled them to stay at home. There is a dilemma in home care; poorly qualified people without education, supervision, or preparation are asked to function independently at a very high level.

Ideally, the perfect provider is a nurse prepared in gerontology at the master's level, with case management skills—someone who can assess needs and provide care at a high level. As we look at health care reform, nurses may become the primary providers of health care. It is up to educators to prepare nurses at an advanced level to manage home care successfully. One English nurse discussed the dilemma of district nurses who would soon have prescriptive privileges and who were looking forward to the task. However, if the English nurses add this task to their already complex position, they need to function at a very high level (Luker & Kenrick, 1992). Another nurse, Ellefson (1992), wrote of the complex role of the community health nurse in Norway. Norwegian nursing officers described themselves as managers in the middle, in a role characterized by conflict and ambiguity. Despite these complaints, in an examination of practice patterns, Hughes and Marcantonio (1992) reported that most home health nurses seem satisfied with their jobs and believe they use their best clinical skills and expertise.

The needs and requirements in home care are monumental. Albrecht (1992) described a Delphi study that listed patient outcomes as the greatest research priority in home health nursing. This study reinforced the results of an earlier study on long-term care (including home care) that also listed knowledge of patient outcomes as the most important need (Haight & Bahr, 1992). Despite the continued cry for outcomes research, the research done on interventions and outcomes in home health care is minimal. Consequently, nurses don't really know what is happening in home care except that they respond to people's needs. Now that we have identified the scope of the problem and the needs of providers, our next effort should be to manage the problem and to apply the knowledge we have.

CASE MANAGEMENT

Initially, the successful home health nurse must be a good manager, particularly if the nurse is to use LPNs and aides to extend professional nursing. The nurse must manage: (1) the client, keeping environment and culture in mind; (2) the family, who also function as caregivers; (3) the personnel (aides and LPNs), who are crucial to delivery of care; and (4) the functional disabilities of the patient, including both physical and psychosocial problems. In addition, the case manager must be aware of available services and helping agencies. Figure 8.2 depicts a case management model that is useful to nurses who take care of the elderly at home (Moxley, 1989). O'Hare and Terry (1991) presented a similar model and spoke of care management rather than case management. In both models, the nurse determines the allocation of resources and, in this way, achieves a needed power.

With case management in place, it is necessary to look at technology as an aid to the work of case management. A patient classification system will help the case manager organize a caseload. With sicker people being discharged to the home, some visits may take longer as the nurse tends to acute-care needs (Churness, Kleffel, & Onodera, 1991). The term "sicker and quicker" aptly describes the hospital discharge process, but sicker and quicker is not the only problem. Many home health nurses experience the Friday dumping syndrome as well. Hospitals clear out their rooms to make way for new admissions over the weekend, never thinking how these discharged older people will function without full services over the weekend.

In addition to these concerns, the home health nurse must be familiar with advanced technology for patient care and record keeping. Not only should the nurse be using a computer to streamline record keeping, but a computer monitor placed in the home can help the patient and family monitor care. For example, if an incisional site became hot and red, the

Figure 8.2
Case Management Model

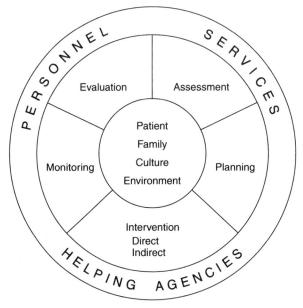

Adapted from *The practice of case management,* by D. Moxley, Sage Human Services Guides (Vol. 58), Newbury Park, CA.

patient could enter this information into a computer and the computer would either tell the patient what to do or tell the patient to come into the office to see the doctor.

Brennan, Moore, and Smyth (1991) described the use of computers by elderly caregivers, who not only received medical information and affirmation, but also communicated with one another on the computer and formed a support group that shared information. An example of this sharing among families with Alzheimer's disease is shown in Figure 8.3. Only two things create a boundary for the use of innovative programs: (1) the imagination of the nurse case manager and (2) funds. Funds may not always be necessary, but imagination always is.

Using volunteers to visit older people at home will extend care and services to a growing number of frail elderly patients. Shugart (1992) described one such program where volunteers were used to provide home care. The American Association of Retired People (AARP) (1989) conducts a similar innovative program using friendly visitors to lead reminiscing programs with homebound elderly people. Reminiscing is particularly enjoyed by those who are homebound and have few people with whom

Figure 8.3
Sharing for Families with Alzheimer's Disease

Question: My husband is in the middle stages of the disease and I would like some suggestions on how to occupy his time other than walking. When he doesn't have anything to do, he seems to want to nap during the day.

Answer: Dorothy I also have a problem with my wife who likes to walk and gets bored! She loves to rearrange her drawers in her dresser! I fix and she rearranges them; it gives her something to do! They always seem to want to be occupied and want to help but it is hard for her! Do your best on this subject.

Adapted from "Computer Link: Electronic Support for the Home Caregiver," by P. F. Brennan, S. M. Moore, & K. A. Smyth. 1991. *Advances in Nursing Science, 13*(4), 14–27.

they can interact (Haight, 1984). Reminiscing programs not only give homebound people an opportunity to talk about the past, they also provide a significant other person who is a good listener. Reminiscence is a way to both *know* about a person and *care* about a person. Other innovative programs reported in nursing journals are: (1) a program that cares for the older person till death at home, not in a hospice (Sweeney, 1988), (2) a team management program for patients with hip fracture (Pryor, Williams, Myles, & Anand, 1988), and (3) provision of nutritional support at home (Orr, 1989).

ENVIRONMENT, CULTURE, AND FAMILY

The nurse who provides care in the patient's home becomes aware of the environment, the culture, and the family; and includes all three in the case management plan. Socioeconomic status often creates the environment, but for many older clients history is just as important to the environment. The patient and his or her family may have been born and raised in a lovely community, but with age this community may have become isolated, unsafe, and without services and transportation. Therefore, as the nurse becomes acquainted with the patient, the nurse must assess both the inside and the outside of the home. This is not a new thought. In *Notes on Nursing*, Florence Nightingale (1859) focused on the environment and said there were five essential points in securing the health of houses: pure air, pure water, effecient drainage, cleanliness, and light.

When the environmental assessment has been completed, the next focus is culture, which is very often a major influence on the patient's compliance or noncompliance. To care for a patient at home, culture must be respected and the impact of the culture must be analyzed in terms of the problem. In 1992, an expert panel of the American Academy of Nursing issued guidelines for culturally competent care, stressing the importance of culture. These guidelines state the need to enhance teaching, research, and the recruitment of students in all cultures and all disenfranchised populations.

The impact of culture is particularly strong when caring for older patients; often, the nurse cannot achieve the set goals unless cultural care is a part of treatment. For example, in South Carolina, many island people still believe in witchcraft. The root doctor is an important person in their health care system and, for an ordinary physician to practice and be effective, the physician must incorporate cultural values and those of the root doctor into the treatment plan.

The third issue surrounding the person at home is family. The nurse must understand the family systems. Often, identifying family systems can be difficult because of the ways in which families are reconfigured today (Brubaker, 1990). Table 8.1 shows some of the reconfigurations that can occur and can result in concerns that may impact on older clients' well-being. The nurse needs to remember that the family is whoever the patient says it is. Supportive relationships can be infinitely more important than blood relationships, and the nurse giving home care needs to respect those relationships.

Aging families may have psychosocial problems that influence the health status of individual family members. The nurse can uncover these problems through family assessment.

Several experts stress the need for a family focus in caring for older people and the need to be aware of the dynamic interactive experience that family care involves (O'Neill & Sorensen, 1991). In an examination of gerontologic textbooks, few chapters were found to be devoted to family. However, with the increase in home care, attention must be paid to the family unit. With a functionally dependent person at home, there is usually a caregiver who is a family member, and both must be treated as a unit. Often, the care will not happen as intended unless the nurse

Table 8.1
Reconfigured Families and Resulting Problems

Configuration	Problems
I. Married	1. Role change 2. Increased sharing
II. Divorced	1. Decreased income 2. Decreased interactions 3. Need for new identity and routines
III. Widowed	1. Grieving and reactive depression 2. Decreased income 3. Possible relocation 4. Decreased support systems and social networks
IV. Remarried	1. Adjustment for children 2. Different financial systems 3. New family configurations

Source: Adapted from "Family Dynamics," by B. K. Haight & K. H. Leech. In M. Stanley & A. Bear (Eds.), *Health promotion in gerontological nursing practice.* In press. Philadelphia: F.A. Davis Co.

also cares for the family caregiver. Sims, Boland, and O'Neill (1992), in describing decision making in home care by family members, likened it to the Benner (1984) framework of novice and expert. Although family members have no professional knowledge, they become experts through their extensive knowledge of the family member who is ill.

FUNCTION

Function may decrease with age. One example of function assessment is Rueben's model, shown in Table 8.2 (Rueben, 1988).

Rueben's model divides activities of daily living (ADLs) into three levels: (1) advanced, (2) instrumental, and (3) basic. Dividing them in this way contributes to defining a patient classification system. People with advanced activities of daily living (AADLs) are not often seen by home health nurses because they are not homebound. They may still have jobs and participate in sports, though they may be in pain after Saturday morning tennis.

Table 8.2
Rueben's Model of Activities of Daily Living (ADLs)

Type	Activity	Need	Effect
AADLs (Advanced)	Job Sports Recreation	Voluntary	1. Decreased self-esteem 2. Worry about future decline
IADLs (Instrumental)	Shop Phone Look Keep house Take medicine Handle finances	Some elective	1. Needs assistance 2. Relocates
BADLs (Basic)	Bathe Dress Toilet Transfer Feed	Mandatory	1. Needs help with personal care

Source: Presented by David Rueben, M.D., Geriatric Assessment Symposium, San Francisco, November 1988. This version adapted from *Nursing Assessment and Diagnosis* by J. Bellack & B. Edlund. 1992. Boston: Jones & Bartlett.

Nurses, however, see elderly persons with losses of instrumental activities of daily living (IADLs). To address these losses (instrumental activity deficits), the nurse case manager needs to find providers of transportation, house cleaning, and yard care. Those with instrumental activity losses may be older people who want to remain at home.

If the elderly person becomes increasingly frail, basic activities of daily living (BADLs) become a major concern. These needs must be met by caregivers or a home health nurse. With a basic activity deficit, the person may become more difficult to care for at home. For example, incontinence can be a major problem for the caregiver and for the person. A home health nurse with a wide knowledge of gerontology and incontinence care can improve the quality of the older person's life. This type of home care, many times, will allow older persons to remain in their own home for longer periods of time.

In examining function, the nurse needs to look at the total person within the complete environment. A prompt list, related to function, provides an excellent way to monitor the effects of functional problems of older people (Runciman, 1989).

With a prompt list, the nurse can easily evaluate each function. If mobility is a problem, the prompt list aids the nurse in the assessment of the person's exact level of function. The list can be a part of the patient's chart; problems can be circled and dated. The list also serves to inform new or substitute nurses of the patient's past condition when they enter the home. An example of a prompt list is given in Table 8.3.

Psychological issues that home care nurses confront are numerous. One major concern that affects many elderly people is loneliness. The effects of loneliness include malnutrition, social isolation, and depression. Many tools are available to the nurse for psychological assessment.

In summary, the nurse who works at home with an older person must have an extremely broad knowledge base. This health nurse must be a connoisseur of knowing and caring (Jenny & Logan, 1992). The nursing care of older people at home demands a gerontology nursing expert whose knowing is grounded in theory and whose caring comes from a compassionate understanding of the value of individuals.

Table 8.3
Example of Prompt List for the Elderly

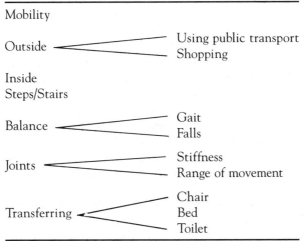

Mobility

Outside — Using public transport / Shopping

Inside
Steps/Stairs

Balance — Gait / Falls

Joints — Stiffness / Range of movement

Transferring — Chair / Bed / Toilet

Source: Adapted from "Health Assessment of the Elderly at Home: The Case for Shared Learning" by P. Runciman. 1989. *Journal of Advanced Nursing, 14,* 111–119.

REFERENCES

AARP. (1989). *Reminiscence: Finding meaning in memories.* Washington, DC: AARP.

Albrecht, M. (1992). Research priorities for home health care nursing. *Nursing & Health Care, 13*(10), 538–541.

Alster, K. B., & Keshian, J. C. (1990). Falling between the cracks: A student experience in providing home care for underserved community-residing elders. *Journal of Community Health Nursing, 7*(1), 15–24.

American Academy of Nursing Expert Panel on Culturally Competent Nursing Care. (1992). AAN expert panel report: Culturally competent health care. *Nursing Outlook, 40*(6), 277–283.

Benner, P. (1984). *From novice to expert: Excellence and power in clinical nursing.* Menlo Park, CA: Addison-Wesley.

Betts, G. (1987). Evaluation of a nursing aide's scheme for elderly people. *Journal of Advanced Nursing, 12,* 85–94.

Brennan, P. F., Moore, S. M., & Smyth, K. A. (1991). ComputerLink: Electronic support for the home caregiver. *Advances in Nursing Science, 13*(4), 14–27.

Brubaker, T. H. (1990). Families in later life: A burgeoning research area. *Journal of Marriage and the Family, 52,* 959.

Churness, V. H., Kleffel, D., & Onodera, M. (1991). Home health patient classification system. *Home Healthcare Nurse, 9*(2), 14–22.

Cudney, S. A. (1992). Bringing gerontic education to rural nurses. *Caring Magazine, 11*(2), 30–35.

Ellefson, B. (1992). The complex role of a community health nurse officer in Norway. *Western Journal of Nursing Research, 14*(2), 142–156.

Haight, B. K., & Bahr, R. T. (1992). Setting an agenda for clinical nursing research in long-term care. *Clinical Nursing Research, 1*(2), 144–157.

Hughes, K. K., & Marcantonio, R. J. (1992). Practice patterns among home health, public health, and hospital nurses. *Nursing & Health Care, 13*(10), 532–536.

Jenny, J., & Logan, J. (1992). Knowing the patient: One aspect of clinical knowledge. *Image: The Journal of Nursing Scholarship, 24*(4), 254–258.

Luker, K. A., & Kenrick, M. (1992). An exploratory study of the sources of influence on the clinical decisions of community nurses. *Journal of Advanced Nursing, 17,* 457–466.

Mitchell, M. K. (1992). CHAP: Nursing's legacy of leadership. *Nursing & Health Care, 13*(6), 296–302.

Moxley, D. (1989). *The practice of case management.* Sage Human Services Guides (Vol. 58). Newbury Park, CA: Sage.

Nightingale, F. (1859). *Notes on nursing.* Philadelphia: Lippincott.

O'Hare, P., & Terry, M. A. (1991). Community-based care management: A Program Resources Department framework for delivery of services. *Home Healthcare Nurse, 9*(3), 26–32.

O'Neill, C., & Sorensen, E. S. (1991). Home care of the elderly: A family perspective. *Advances in Nursing Science, 13*(4), 28–37.

Orr, M. E. (1989). Nutritional support in home care. *Advances in Nutritional Support, 24*(2), 437–445.

Pryor, G. A., Williams, D. R. R., Myles, J. W., & Anand, J. K. (1988). Team management of the elderly patient with hip fracture. *The Lancet, 1*(8582), 401–403.

Rueben, D. (1988). *Rueben's model of activity.* Geriatric Assessment Symposium, San Francisco, November 1988.

Runciman, P. (1989). Health assessment of the elderly at home: The case for shared learning. *Journal of Advanced Nursing, 14,* 111–119.

Savorgnani, A., Haring, R. C., & Galloway, S. (1992). Caught in the middle: A profile of licensed practical nurses in home care. *Caring Magazine, 11*(9), 12–16.

Sims, S. L., Boland, D. L., & O'Neill, C. A. (1992). Decision making in home health care. *Western Journal of Nursing Research, 14*(2), 186–200.

Sweeney, J. M. (1988). Let him go home! *Geriatric Nursing, 9*(6), 344–346.

Shugart, E. B. (1992). Using volunteer visitors in home care. *Journal of Nursing Administration, 22*(4), 42–45.

U. S. Department of Health & Human Services. (1992a). *The noninstitutionalized elderly: Ability to perform daily activities* (AHCPR Report No. 7). Rockville, MD: Agency for Health Care Policy and Research (AHCPR Publication No. 92-0106).

U. S. Department of Health & Human Services. (1992b). *The noninstitutionalized elderly: Characteristics of persons with functional limitations.* (AHCPR Report No. 8.) Rockville, MD: Agency for Health Care Policy and Research (AHCPR Publication No. 92-0107).

U. S. Department of Health & Human Services. (1992c). *The elderly with functional difficulties: Patterns of use of home and community services.* (AHCPR Report No. 12.) Rockville, MD: Agency for Health Care Policy and Research (AHCPR Publication No. 92-0111).

9

Quality of Caring:
The Elderly at Home

Linda R. Phillips

When quality of caring for the elderly is discussed, the focus automatically fixes on the quality of care in institutional settings. Although the quality of institutional care is important, it is a very small part of the problem of assuring quality care to the elderly.

According to a growing national data base (e.g., Branch & Jette, 1983; Brody, 1985; Brody, Kleban, Johnsen, Hoffman, & Schoonover, 1987; Brody & Schoonover, 1986; Cantor, 1983; Doty, 1986; Horowitz & Dobrof, 1982; Liu, Manton, & Liu, 1985; Moss, Moos, & Moles, 1985; Noelker & Poulshock, 1982; Select Committee on Aging, 1987; Shanas, 1979; Stephens & Christianson, 1986; Stone, Carrerate, & Sangi, 1987; Tennstedt & McKinlay, 1989), most elders do not live in institutions. Regardless of the elder's health, the intensity of need, family members' other responsibilities, whether or not the elder lives alone, the geographic closeness of family members, and the family's ethnic/cultural background, most elders live at home and, if needed, receive care in that setting.

Without a doubt, family members provide the bulk of long-term care to elders in this country. Without the care provided to elders by family members, our country's long-term care resources would be overwhelmed by the needs. Improving the quality of care provided to the elderly in this country is dependent on understanding and developing strategies for improving the quality of in-home caring, including the care provided by family members.

The quality of in-home caring for the elderly is very complex; it involves structural and interpersonal aspects. Structurally, in-home care involves many discrete service delivery systems that vary by capacity for external regulation, amount of formalization, and organization. There is no uniform financing and almost no uniform organization (Evashwick, 1985). To say the least, the interrelationships among structures are intricate. In addition, most home care is delivered by the informal service delivery structure, for which almost no external regulatory mechanisms exist.

The interpersonal aspects of in-home caring involve intrafamily dynamics, intra-agency dynamics, and the linkages among elders, family members, and agency personnel. To further complicate the picture, few alternatives to care at home exist that are *acceptable* to either elders or family members. Institutional long-term care has never been philosophically appealing to either elders or families in the United States. In addition, under the current reimbursement system, institutional placement is not a viable option for most families.

From a nursing perspective, quality of in-home caring for the elderly is particularly complicated. In formal home care agencies, nurses are accountable for the quality of the care, even though they do not actually provide the bulk of the care themselves. In the home, nurses often serve in educational/advisory capacities, and actual care is provided by either family caregivers or nonprofessional staff. Some care that family members provide is highly technical, and the family is expected to provide care largely unassisted and with relatively little training. In light of the demographic patterns, a large proportion of family caregivers are spouses or adult children who are themselves over the age of 65 and facing chronic health problems. This presents special dilemmas for the evaluation of quality indicators.

To further complicate the picture, regulatory standards coupled with cost incentives serve to limit the amount of involvement of professional nurses in home care. To illustrate, although a portion of the elders who are discharged to home receive home health visits early in their recovery (the national average is 30 visits (Harrington, 1987)), if their recuperation is prolonged or if their disease is chronic, the only help likely to be available is that paid for out-of-pocket. Usually, such care is *not* provided by professional nurses. If the elder has not had an acute illness requiring hospitalization, the types of services available to the family are even more limited and the likelihood of care from a professional nurse is even less.

In the home, the quality of care can only be ensured to the degree that the nurse can mobilize others to meet quality criteria. For some elders, this is a minor problem; their informal home care is supportive and adequate to meet their needs. For others, the picture is different. A growing body of research suggests that the quality of informal home care varies widely. Increasingly, research indicates: (1) the quality of care for some elders is less than optimal, resulting in unmet physical, emotional, and social needs; and (2) some elders are at high risk for abuse, neglect, and other forms of maltreatment by their informal care providers (Giordano & Giordano, 1983; Hickey & Douglass, 1981a, 1981b; Lau & Kosberg, 1979; O'Malley, Everitt, O'Malley, & Campion, 1983; Phillips, 1983; Pillemer, 1985, 1986; Pillemer & Finkelhor, 1988; Steinmetz, 1981; Wolf, Godkin, & Pillemer, 1984). Differentiating between elders whose care is adequate and elders whose care is poor or abusive can be very problematic because definitions of quality of care are not firmly established and few standards exist on which the quality of family care can be evaluated.

Given this background, this chapter will focus on the issues involved in applying quality standards to the available formal and informal care systems for providing in-home care to elders. For the purpose of this chapter, quality of care is defined as the degree or grade of excellence displayed in attempting to meet the needs of dependent elders at home (adapted from Wandelt & Stewart, 1975). Quality of care is conceptualized as a continuum that ranges from excellence to abuse/neglect.

QUALITY STANDARDS FOR HOME CARE SYSTEMS

Various standards for evaluating the quality of health care services have been developed. In 1968, for example, Donabedian stated standards for evaluating the quality of health services needed to focus on the structures, processes, and outcomes of care. Aday and Andersen (1975) recommended access, acceptability, and availability as the criteria necessary for evaluating the quality of community-based services. Evashwick (1988) proposed, regarding community-based services, that attention to between-service components was essential to evaluating quality. Therefore, standards needed to include:

1. The client's access to appropriate services at appropriate times;
2. Monitoring of the client's condition and changing services as needs change;

3. Coordination among many professionals and disciplines;
4. Integration of a range of settings into the care plan;
5. Matching of resources to the client's condition in a efficient and cost-effective manner.

Standards for evaluating the quality of long-term care in institutions have also been discussed in the literature. For example, the Institute of Medicine (IOM) (1986) stated: "The attributes of quality in nursing homes are very different from those in acute medical care settings such as hospitals" (p. 45). The difference stems from:

1. Characteristics of residents' care needs;
2. The circumstances and settings in which care is provided;
3. The expected outcomes;
4. The fact that, for many, the nursing home is their home, not a temporary placement experience. (IOM, 1986)

Expectation for achievement among nursing home residents is low, and few ever leave or return to a lower level of care (Savinshinsky, 1992). Residents often have a poor prognosis (Phillips, 1987) and require the most basic care, and death is a relatively common occurrence (Woods & Britton, 1985). These observations about institutional long-term care are also applicable to long-term care in the home: they suggest outcome criteria for evaluating quality are different for long-term care versus acute care.

Standards for evaluating the quality of home care have also been discussed in the literature; however, the focus has been primarily on evaluating the care provided by professionals or nonprofessional staff (e.g., Daniels, 1986; Mumma, 1987). Methods for evaluating care provided by families have received limited attention.

In this discussion, the standards to be applied to available home care systems are: *structure, process, access, outcomes,* and *dynamics.* In addition, in-home services have both "macro" and "micro" elements. Overall, the macro element involves the organizational unit of analysis. Quality assurance, for example, focuses on the macro elements and has been largely defined by the degree to which formal agencies (e.g., extended care facilities, skilled nursing facilities) adhere to regulations concerning licensing, certification, and staff ratios. The micro level focuses on the individual unit of analysis and seeks to ascertain the degree to which the system and the care providers representing the system respond to the needs of individual care recipients. Both macro and micro elements will be addressed in this discussion.

Structure

When institutional long-term care is discussed, structure includes such factors as nursing home size (Kart & Manard, 1976; Penchansky & Taubenhaus, 1965; Riportella-Muller & Slesinger, 1982; Tobin, 1974), patient-to-staff ratios, and organizational characteristics (Epstein, 1981; Gottesman & Bourestom, 1974; Greenwald & Linn, 1971; Linn, 1966; 1974). For in-home care, structure involves some of the same factors plus consideration of types of systems, organization of systems, and interrelationships among systems.

Home care has both formal and informal aspects (Figure 9.1). Formal home care consists of health and/or social services provided by paid staff to individuals and families in their homes or other community and home-like settings. Formal home care involves an array of nursing, rehabilitation, social work, home health aid, and other types of services. It can involve short- and long-term services designed to supplement, complement, or substitute for institutional care. Short-term home care usually focuses on intermittent care after a hospital discharge. Long-term home care can augment other services provided to the elder or may be a substitute for

Figure 9.1
Applying Quality Standards to Available
Home Care Systems

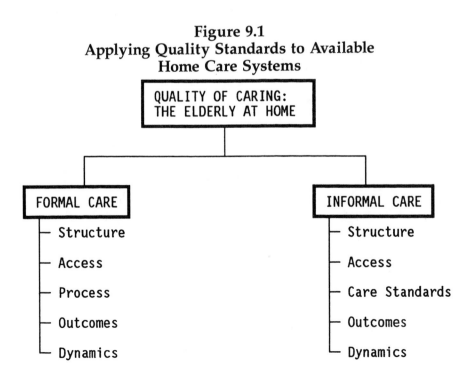

nursing home or hospital care. Harrington, et al. (1988) described six basic types of formal home care service providers:

1. Licensed-only, noncertified home health agencies;
2. Licensed and certified home health agencies;
3. Nurses' registries;
4. Employment agencies;
5. Unlicensed or temporary personnel agencies;
6. Public contract providers.

Informal home care is health and/or social services provided to elders and families in the community by unpaid nonprofessionals, including family members, friends, and neighbors. Like formal home care, informal home care can be short-term or long-term, intermittent or constant. It may supplement formal services or be the only services provided. It may substitute for nursing home or hospital care.

Evaluating the structure of formal home care involves attention to the types of home care available, sources of payment, duration of care, supervision of personnel, services offered, and payment arrangements. Evaluating the informal caregiving structure involves consideration of the family or network structure, the historical context of the structure, the structure of the role relationships, socioeconomic status, and culture-ethnicity. Factors to be considered include the intergenerational arrangements, gender of providers and gender-specific role definitions, family norms (including norms of obligation and solidarity), power structure among members, and role proscriptions for network members (Phillips, 1989).

Process

Process measures take into account conformance to standards and regulatory codes, and ratings by consumers (Riportella-Muller & Slesinger, 1982). Evaluation of care processes is based on the assumption that accepted standards exist. For formal home care, standards exist in the form of regulatory codes, including Medicaid and Medicare regulations and state regulations. In addition, formal home care agencies, if run by professionals, adhere to the professional standards of excellence of the various professions involved.

For informal home care, standards of care have yet to be firmly established, but it is clear that standards vary based on whose opinion is considered (e.g., care recipient, informal caregiver, formal caregiver). Even within groups, opinions can vary. Satisfaction with care is often used as a standard for elders. Satisfaction, however, is a "slippery" indicator. For example, for some elders, satisfaction may be based on a standard of excellence that dictates maintaining autonomy. If this is the case, satisfaction is expressed only when the caregiver restricts caregiving activities to instances when the elder is unable to meet personal needs. For other elders, however, satisfaction may be based on a standard of excellence that involves the caregiver's meeting a majority of their needs regardless of their physical status. For these elders, relinquishing control to experts or responsible persons leads to satisfaction. Client satisfaction is an important aspect of evaluating the quality of caregiving, but many nurses question whether patients have the knowledge to accurately evaluate the technical aspects of care (Cromwell et al., 1993). In addition, satisfaction is always mediated by expectations. As a result, an individual can be very satisfied with poor care if he or she expects nothing more or has no other standards for comparison.

Family caregivers also have standards for quality of care, even though these standards have been little studied. Bowers' (1987) research provided an examination of how family caregivers' standards for quality of caregiving differ from those of health professionals. In her study, family caregivers indicated that protecting the elder's self-image from the possible negative consequences of his or her behavior (protective caregiving) was the most important type of caregiving. This was in contrast to the preventive and instrumental caregiving most highly valued by health care professionals.

Standards from authoritative experts (Chance, 1980), such as health professionals, can also be used in a process evaluation of informal caregiving. For example, one approach to deriving a standard for quality of elder caregiving uses elders' perceived quality of life as an indicator of quality of care. Quality of life indicators, such as elder morale (e.g., Ryden, 1984) and psychological well being (e.g., Bowser, 1987) are sometimes useful standards for evaluating the processes of informal caregiving. These standards are greatly influenced by the ethical and moral values of the professionals deriving the standards, leading to a criterion of adequacy rather than excellence, and often do not take into account cultural variation (Cromwell et al., 1993). Defining quality as adequacy only establishes the lower bound for acceptable care based on expert judgments and may, in fact, be insensitive to cultural differences.

One resolution to this dilemma is the use of standards of excellence for informal caregiving based on basic human rights (Phillips, Morrison, & Chae, 1990). The precedent for such standards of excellence rests in the United Nations Universal Declaration of Human Rights, which contains definitions of both the civil/political rights and the economic/social/cultural rights of all human beings (General Assembly of the United Nations, 1948). For example, Article 25 of this document states every human being has the right to "a standard of living adequate for the health and well-being of himself and his family, including food, clothing, housing and medical care . . . necessary social services, . . . the right to security in the event of sickness, disability, . . . (or) old age . . ." (General Assembly of the United Nations, 1948). In general, these standards apply irrespective of the nationality or cultural/ethnic background of the individuals involved, but the ways in which the standards are operationalized can vary within and between cultures (Cromwell et al., 1993).

Examples of how universal standards of human rights can be used to evaluate quality of informal caregiving are found in the work of Phillips et al. (1990). The United Nations Universal Declaration of Human Rights indicates all humans have the right to (1) a safe environment, (2) physical well-being, (3) health care, (4) psychosocial well-being, (5) choices, and (6) access to resources and assets. These can be directly observed in caregiving situations. For example, evidence of a safe environment would include assurance that the elder's sleeping space is clean and adequate and the elder's residence is safe from burglary, and so on. Evidence of physical well-being would include assurance that the caregiver regularly attends to the elder's personal hygiene needs, the elder's need for exercise and movement, and the elder's need for attire that is adequate for the environment, activity level, and so on.

In summary, whether formal or informal caregiving is being evaluated, process evaluation rests on the assumption that formal standards exist and the grade of excellence can be identified based on the degree to which standards are met. In fact, some standards do exist for evaluation of formal caregiving processes. For informal caregiving, however, no firm standards exist, and application of any standards is complicated by the great variation that exists among data sources.

Access

Access is the degree to which individuals perceive services are available for their use. For formal caregiving, access is influenced by at least two factors: (1) the rurality of the caregiving situation, and (2) the knowledge of health professionals. In general, rural elders have the same acute-care needs as urban elders, but services available in rural areas are far fewer. As a whole, rural elders must depend on family caregivers to a much greater extent than their urban counterparts, because of a lack of services of all types and long-term care services in particular. The degree to which rurality influences the quality of in-home care to the elderly is not known, but elders in rural setting clearly have far fewer options for care than do urban elders.

Even in urban areas, access to in-home care is greatly influenced by the knowledge of health care professionals. All possible services can be available, but if gatekeepers such as primary care physicians are not knowledgeable about availability and eligibility or are insensitive to needs other than acute medical needs as evidenced during an office visit, access to services will be greatly limited. Acute-care facilities that have no formal mechanisms for identifying high-risk elders and referring such elders to formal services also contribute to the lack of access. If formal in-home services were well-organized and standardized across communities, the problem would not be especially acute. However, given the unorganized and unstandardized nature of formal in-home services, access is ensured only to the degree that elders and families are provided help in negotiating the service delivery maze.

For informal caregiving, access is influenced by (1) family characteristics, including education and sophistication; (2) the presenting health care problems; and (3) the availability of other social support. Families vary greatly in their abilities to identify when institution of caregiving relationships is necessary. This is particularly true when the deterioration of the elder is slow and no catastrophic problem brings the need for care to the family's immediate attention (Phillips, 1991). Although families' willingness to provide care is not influenced by ethnicity or geographic distance from the elder, it is most likely influenced by family members' knowledge about aging, the expectations family members share regarding appropriate behavioral expressions of the aging experience, and the organization of the family with regard to an identified and identifiable primary caregiver (Phillips, 1991). Coupled with the nature of presenting health problems and the size and density of the support network, these factors influence the access of an elder to informal in-home caregiving.

Outcomes

Outcomes are the degree to which care yields positive results. Evaluating care outcomes is a common, popular approach to judging quality.

For elders in the home, however, identifying appropriate outcomes is complicated, whether the care is provided by the formal or informal service sector. Traditional outcome indicators include functional/behavioral decline, stability, affect, and service utilization. Although all of these are appropriate to some degree, the issue is far from simple because, with the elderly, some decline and change in affect over time are expected and some chronic disease trajectories are not stable, regardless of the quality of care. Outcome measures for in-home care need to take these complications into consideration. Potentially fruitful areas for examining outcomes for elders at home may be concepts such as goal attainment and prevention of induced dependency and premature decline. Such indicators may more fairly indicate quality outcome than the traditional indicators commonly used.

Dynamics

Dynamics involves the ways systems and subsystems interact. For formal in-home caregiving, dynamics involves the interactions among and between agencies and the interactions among and between individuals, including the elder and family with agencies and agency personnel. Key issues in evaluating dynamics are those involving the ways in which: (1) care is coordinated, (2) changes in condition and care transitions (e.g., from home to hospital and back) are managed, (3) resources are matched to need, and (4) day-to-day interactions influence the acceptability and use of services. Reluctance of elders and caregivers to use some types of services (e.g., respite) despite availability is well-documented. The ways in which services are organized (e.g., hours of operation, rules for use) and the interpretation elders and caregivers give their responsibility for service use (e.g., perceived need to clean before the cleaning woman comes) are factors in the reluctance to use services. Perceived barriers to service use are key factors in evaluating the dynamics of care.

For informal caring, dynamics involves the nature of the interactions between elders and family members, among family members and between family members and the health care systems. Key issues in evaluating informal caregiving dynamics are the ways in which: (1) care eliciting and care receiving are proscribed within the family system and (2) care work is distributed and negotiated among family members. Understanding how care providers view their roles and integrate these roles into their daily lives is essential for evaluating the way in which caregiving dynamics influences the outcomes of care.

ISSUES IN APPLYING QUALITY STANDARDS

In summary, the following issues apply to assessing the quality of in-home care.

- Evaluation of the quality of in-home care needs to consider care provided by the formal sector and care provided by the informal sector. The factors that need to be considered for both types of care include structure, process, access, outcomes, and dynamics. Both macro-level and micro-level evaluations are important. Many of the factors that affect quality of formal in-home care also affect the quality of informal care. Formal and informal care are intimately related, and problems in one sector intensify problems of the other. Therefore, it is impossible to fairly assess the quality of in-home care without considering the quality of formal care, the quality of informal care, and the interrelationships between the two.

- The attributes of quality in the home are different from those in other settings. The differences stem from: (1) the characteristics of elders' care needs, (2) the setting and circumstances of care, (3) the expected outcomes of care, (4) the nature of other alternatives available for care, and (5) social imperatives that dictate home care is more desirable than other care alternatives. The difference in attributes influences the factors that are appropriate to evaluate and the nature of the standards applied.

- The match between resources and the elder's condition is critical for evaluating the quality of in-home care, including (1) access to appropriate services at the appropriate times and (2) the problems of service fragmentation and lack of provider information. In no other setting are the care coordination and communication during changes in client condition and care transitions more critical to consider.

- At a point, regardless of the services in play, there is no caregiving without *caregivers*. Therefore, targeting formal services only to elders without considering the needs of the caregivers is counterproductive. Evaluations of quality must include consideration of the degree to which the needs of the elder are met and the degree to which the needs of the caregivers are met. In addition, unlike care provided in hospitals, care outcomes in the home rely primarily on the skills and expertise of family members and/or paid nonprofessionals and secondarily on the counseling and educational roles of nurses.

All of these are crucial considerations in formal evaluations of the quality of in-home services for the elderly.

REFERENCES

Aday, L., & Andersen, R. (1975). *Access to medical care*. Ann Arbor, MI: Health Administration Press.

Bowers, B. (1987). Intergenerational caregiving: Adult caregivers and their aging parents. *Advances in Nursing Science, 9*(2), 20–3.

Bowser, J. (1987). Personal control and psychological well-being of institutionalized elders. *Dissertation Abstracts, 48*(5), 1299B.

Branch, L., & Jette, A. (1983). Elder's use of informal long-term care assistance. *The Gerontologist, 23*, 51–56.

Brody, E. (1985). Parent care as a normative family stress. *The Gerontologist, 25*, 19–29.

Brody, E., Kleban, M., Johnsen, P., Hoffman, C., & Schoonover, C. (1987). Work status and parent care: A comparison of four groups of women. *The Gerontologist, 27*, 201–208.

Brody, E., & Schoonover, C. (1986). Patterns of parent care when adult daughters work and when they do not. *The Gerontologist, 26*, 372–382.

Cantor, M. (1983). Strain among caregivers: A study of experience in the United States. *The Gerontologist, 23*, 597–604.

Chance, K. (1980). The quest for quality: An exploration of attempts to define and measure quality nursing care. *Image: The Journal of Nursing Scholarship, 12*(2), 41–45.

Cromwell, S., Russell, C., Chae, Y., Luna, I., Torres de Ardon, E., & Phillips, L. (1993). Uncovering the cultural context for quality of family caregiving for the elderly. Unpublished manuscript. University of Arizona, Tucson.

Daniels, K. (1986). Planning for quality in the home care system. *QRB, 12*(7), 247–251.

Donabedian, A. (1968). Promoting quality through evaluating process of care. *Medical Care, 6*(3), 181–202.

Doty, P. (1986). Family care of the elderly: The role of public policy. *Milbank Memorial Fund Quarterly, 64*, 34–75.

Epstein, W. (1981). A comparison between the Veterans Administration's long-term care nursing home care program and three examples of similar care outside of the VA. *International Journal of Aging and Human Development, 13*, 61–69.

Evashwick, (1985). Home health care current trends and future opportunities. *Journal of Ambulatory Care Management, 8*(4), 4–17.

General Assembly of the United Nations (1948). Universal Declaration of Human Rights. In *The New Encyclopedia Britannica,* 15th edition (1986). Chicago: Encyclopedia Britannica.

Giordano, N., & Giordano, J. (1983, November). *Individual and family correlates of elder abuse.* Unpublished paper presented at the 36th Annual Scientific Meeting of the Gerontology Society of America, San Francisco.

Gottesman, L., & Bourestom, N. (1974). Why nursing homes do what they do. *The Gerontologist, 14,* 501–506.

Greenwald, S., & Linn, M. (1971). Intercorrelation of data on nursing homes. *The Gerontologist, 11,* 337–330.

Harrington, C. (1987). Nursing home reform: Addressing critical staffing issues. *Nursing Outlook, 35,* 208–209.

Harrington, et al. (1988). Quality, access and costs: Public policy and home health care. *Nursing Outlook, 36*(4), 164–166.

Hickey, T., & Douglass, R. L. (1981a). The mistreatment of the elderly in the domestic setting: An exploratory study. *American Journal of Public Health, 71,* 500–507.

Hickey, T., & Douglass, R. L. (1981b). Neglect and abuse of older family members: Professionals' perspectives and care experiences. *The Gerontologist, 21,* 171–176.

Horowitz, A., & Dobrof, R. (1982). *The role of families in providing long-term care to the frail and chronically ill elderly living in the community.* Final report submitted to Health Care Financing Administration. New York: Brookdale Center on Aging.

Institute of Medicine. (1986). *Improving the quality of care in nursing homes.* Washington, DC: National Academy Press.

Kart, C., & Manard, B. (1976). Quality of care in old age institutions. *The Gerontologist, 16,* 250–256.

Lau, E., & Kosberg, J. (1979). Abuse of the elderly by informal care providers. *Aging, 299,* 10–15.

Linn, M. (1966). A nursing home rating scale. *Geriatrics, 21,* 188–192.

Linn, M. (1974). Predicting the quality of patient care in nursing homes. *The Gerontologist, 14,* 225–227.

Liu, K., Manton, K., & Liu, B. (1985). Home care expenses for noninstitutionalized elderly with ADL and IADL limitations. *Health Care Financing Review, 7,* 51–58.

Moss, M., Moos, S., & Moles, E. (1985). The relationship between elderly parents and their out-of-town children. *The Gerontologist, 25,* 134–140.

Mumma, N. L. (1987). Quality and cost control of home care services through coordinated funding. *QRB. 13*(8), 271–278.

Noelker, L., & Poulshock, S. (1982). *The effects on families caring for impaired elderly in residence.* Final report submitted to the Administration on Aging.

Cleveland, OH: Margaret Blenkner Research Center for Family Studies, Benjamin Rose Institute.

O'Malley, T., Everitt, D., O'Malley, H., & Campion, E. (1983). Identifying and preventing abuse and neglect of elderly persons. *Annals of Internal Medicine, 98,* 998–1005.

Penchansky, R., & Taubenhaus, L. (1965). Institutional factors affecting the quality of care in nursing homes. *Geriatrics, 20,* 591–598.

Phillips, C. (1987). Staff turnover in nursing homes for the aged: A review and research proposal. *International Journal of Nursing Studies, 24,* 45–57.

Phillips, L. (1983). Abuse and neglect of the frail elderly at home: An exploration of theoretical relationships. *Journal of Advanced Nursing, 8,* 379–392.

Phillips, L. R. (1989). Elder–family caregiver relationships: Determining appropriate nursing interventions (pp. 795–807). In R. Rempusheski (Ed.), *Nursing clinics of North America.* Philadelphia: Saunders.

Phillips, L. R. (1991). Social supports of the older client. In W. C. Chenitz, J. T. Stone, & S. A. Salisbury (Eds.), *Clinical gerontological nursing* (pp. 535–544). Philadelphia: Saunders.

Phillips. L. R., Morrison, E., & Chae, Y. (1990). The QUALCARE scale: Developing an instrument to measure quality of home care. *International Journal of Nursing Studies, 21,* 61–75.

Pillemer, K. (1985). The dangers of dependency: New findings on domestic violence against the elderly. *Social Problems, 33,* 146–158.

Pillemer, K. (1986). Risk factors in elder abuse: Results of a case-control study. In K. Pillemer & R. Wolf (Eds.), *Elder abuse: Conflict in the family.* Dover, MA: Auburn House.

Pillemer, K., & Finkelhor, D. (1988). Prevalence of elderly abuse: A random sample survey. *The Gerontologist, 28,* 51–57.

Riportella-Muller, R., & Slesinger, D. (1982). The relationship between ownership and size to quality of care in Wisconsin nursing homes. *The Gerontologist, 22,* 429–434.

Ryden, M. (1984). Morale and perceived control in institutionalized elderly. *Nursing Research, 33*(3), 130–136.

Select Committee on Aging. (1987). *Exploding the myths: Caregiving in America.* A study by the Subcommittee on Human Services of the Select Committee on Aging, House of Representatives. Comm. Pub. No. 99-611.

Shanas, E. (1979). Social myth as hypothesis: The case of the family relationships of old people. *The Gerontologist, 19,* 3–9.

Steinmetz, S. (1981). Elder abuse. *Aging, 315–316,* 6–10.

Stephens, S., & Christianson, J. (1986). *Informal care of the elderly.* Lexington, MA: Lexington Books.

Stone, R., Carrerate, G., & Sangi, H. (1987). Caregivers of the frail elderly: A national profile. *The Gerontologist, 27,* 616–626.

Tennestedt, S., & McKinlay, J. (1989). Informal care for frail older persons. In M. Ory & K. Bond (Eds.), *Aging and health care* (pp. 145–166). London: Routledge & Kegan Paul.

Tobin, S. (1974). How nursing homes vary. *The Gerontologist, 14,* 516–519.

Wandelt, M., & Stewart, D. (1975). *Slater Nursing Competency Rating Scale.* New York: Appleton-Century-Crofts.

Wolf, R., Godkin, M., & Pillemer, K. (1984). *Elder abuse and neglect: Final report from three model projects.* Worcester: University of Massachusetts, Medical Center and University Center on Aging. (ERIC Document Reproduction Service No. ED 254796.)

Woods, R., & Britton, P. (1985). *Clinical psychology with the elderly.* Rockville, MD: Aspen Publications.

Other Books of Interest from NLN Press

Book Title	Pub. No.	Price	NLN Member Price
☐ Gerontological Nursing: Issues and Opportunities for the Twenty-First Century *By Mary M. Burke and Susan Sherman*	14-2510	$27.95	$24.95
☐ Determining the Future of Gerontological Nursing Education: Partnerships between Education and Practice *Edited by Christine Heine*	14-2508	26.95	23.95
☐ Teaching Gerontology: The Curriculum Imperative *Edited by Verle Waters*	15-2411	28.95	25.95
☐ Mechanisms of Quality in Long-Term Care: Education *Edited by Ethel L. Mitty*	14-2550	25.95	22.95
☐ Quality Imperatives in Long-Term Care: The Elusive Agenda *Edited by Ethel L. Mitty*	41-2440	25.95	22.95
☐ Gerontology in the Nursing Curriculum *From the Community College/Nursing Home Partnership*	14-2506	6.95	5.95